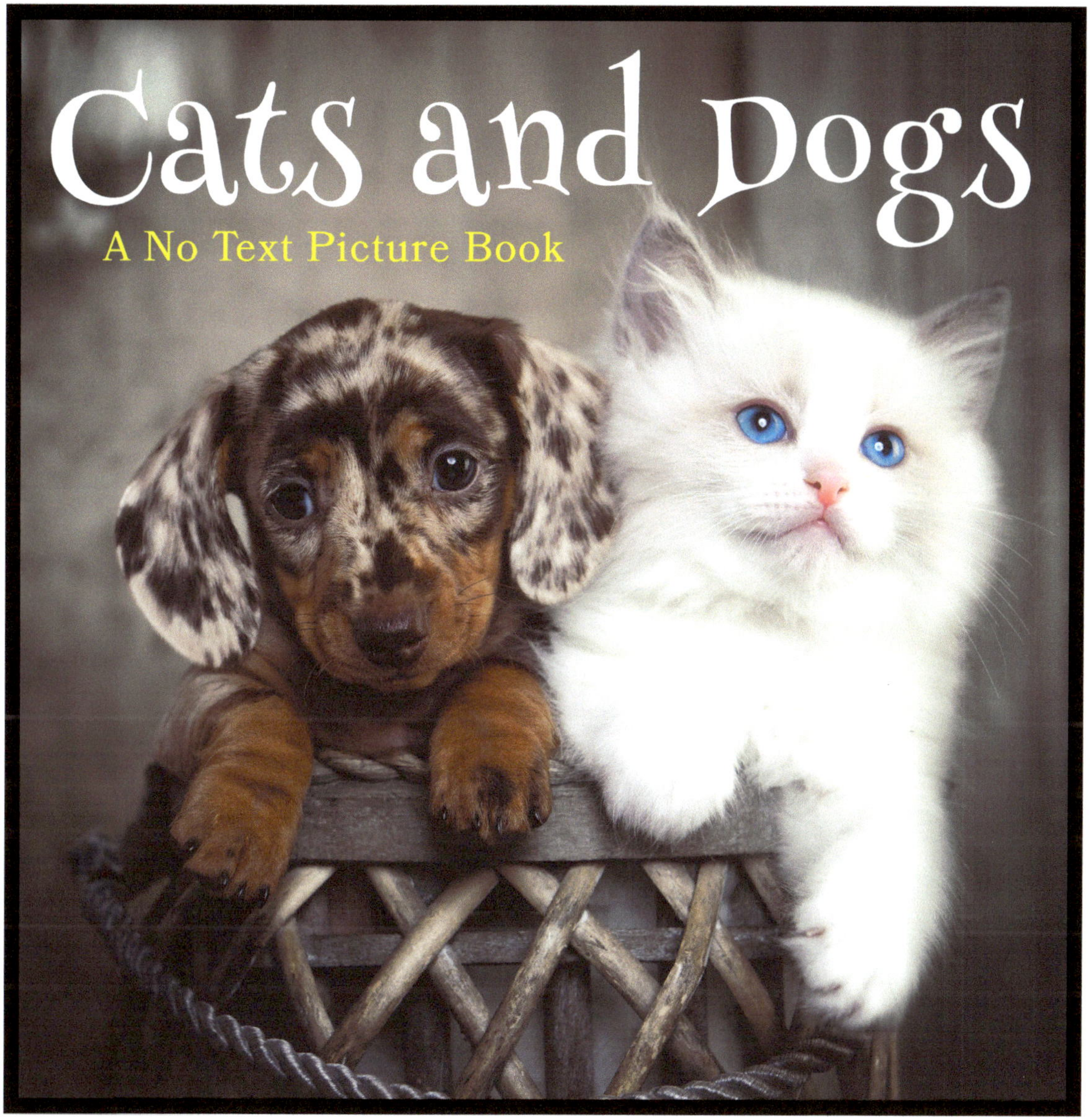

Lasting Happiness

ISBN: 978-1-990181-70-2

To:

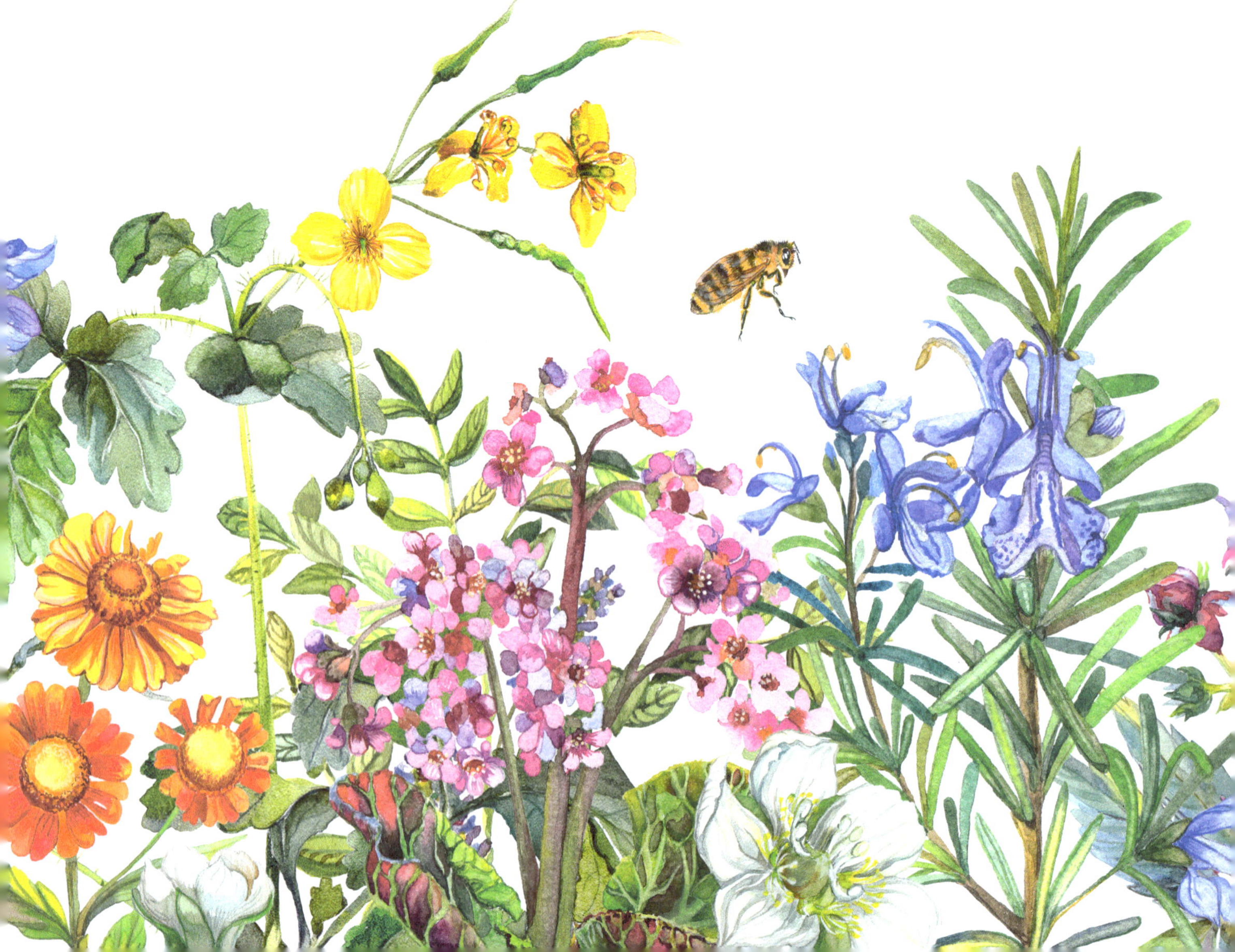

FROM:

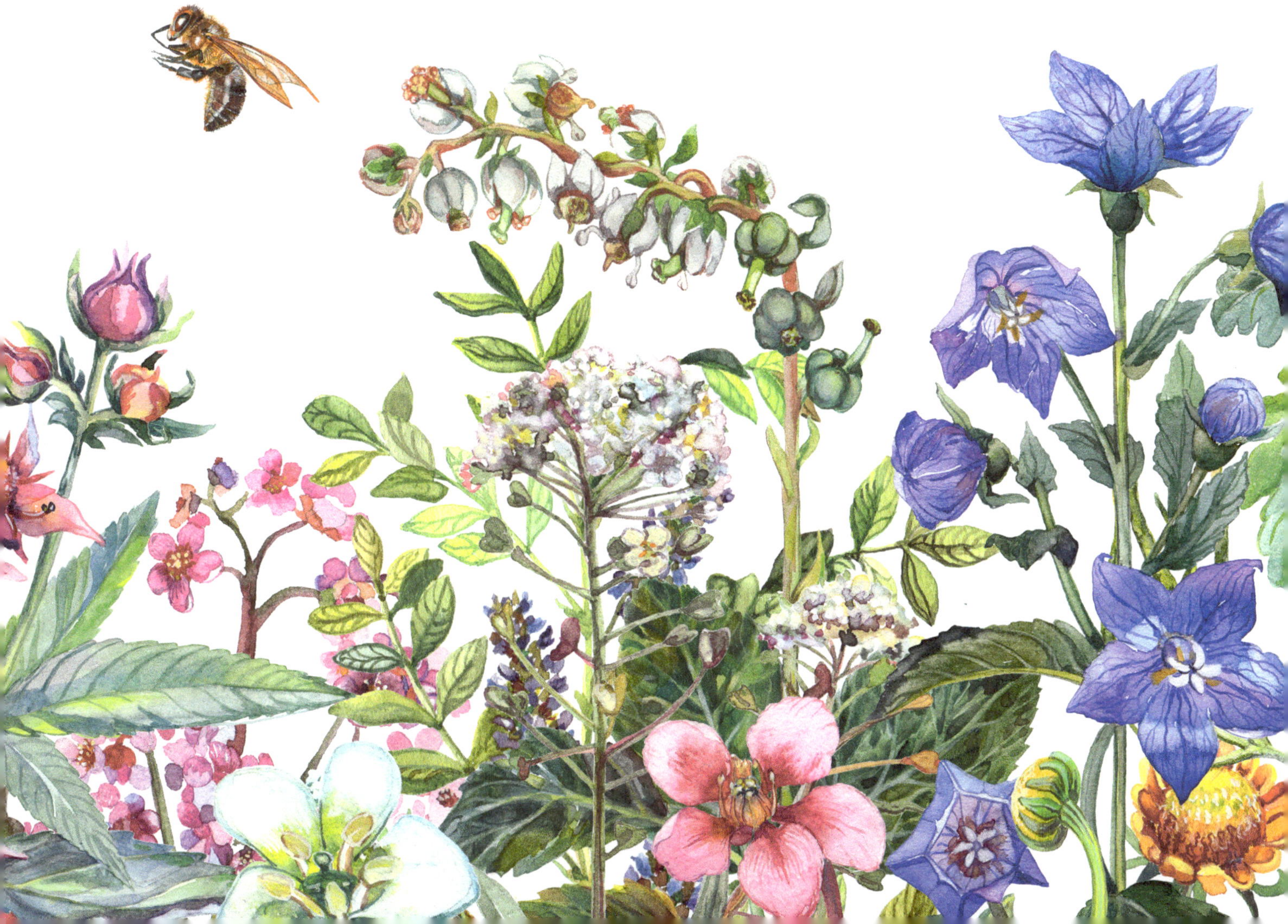

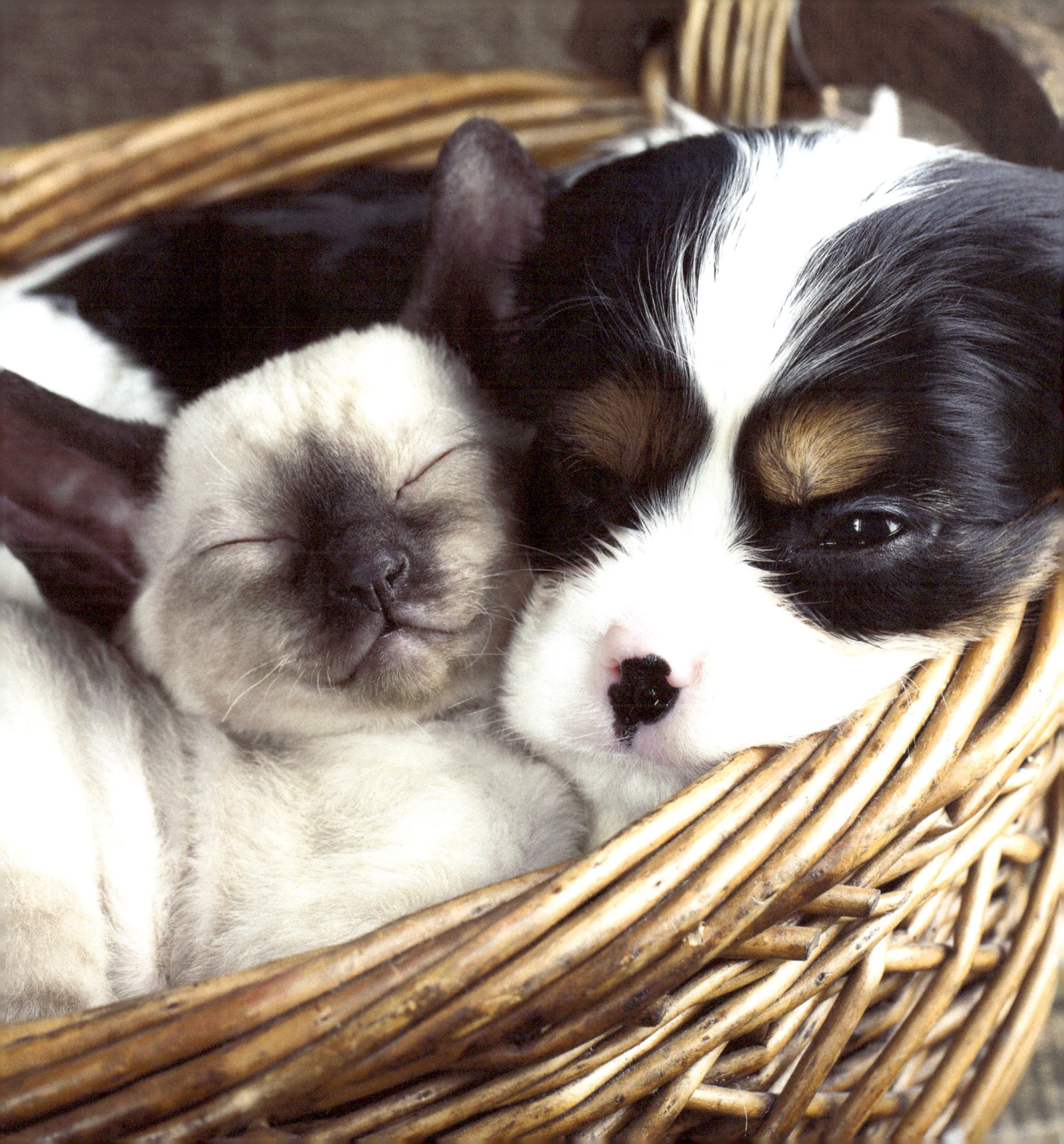

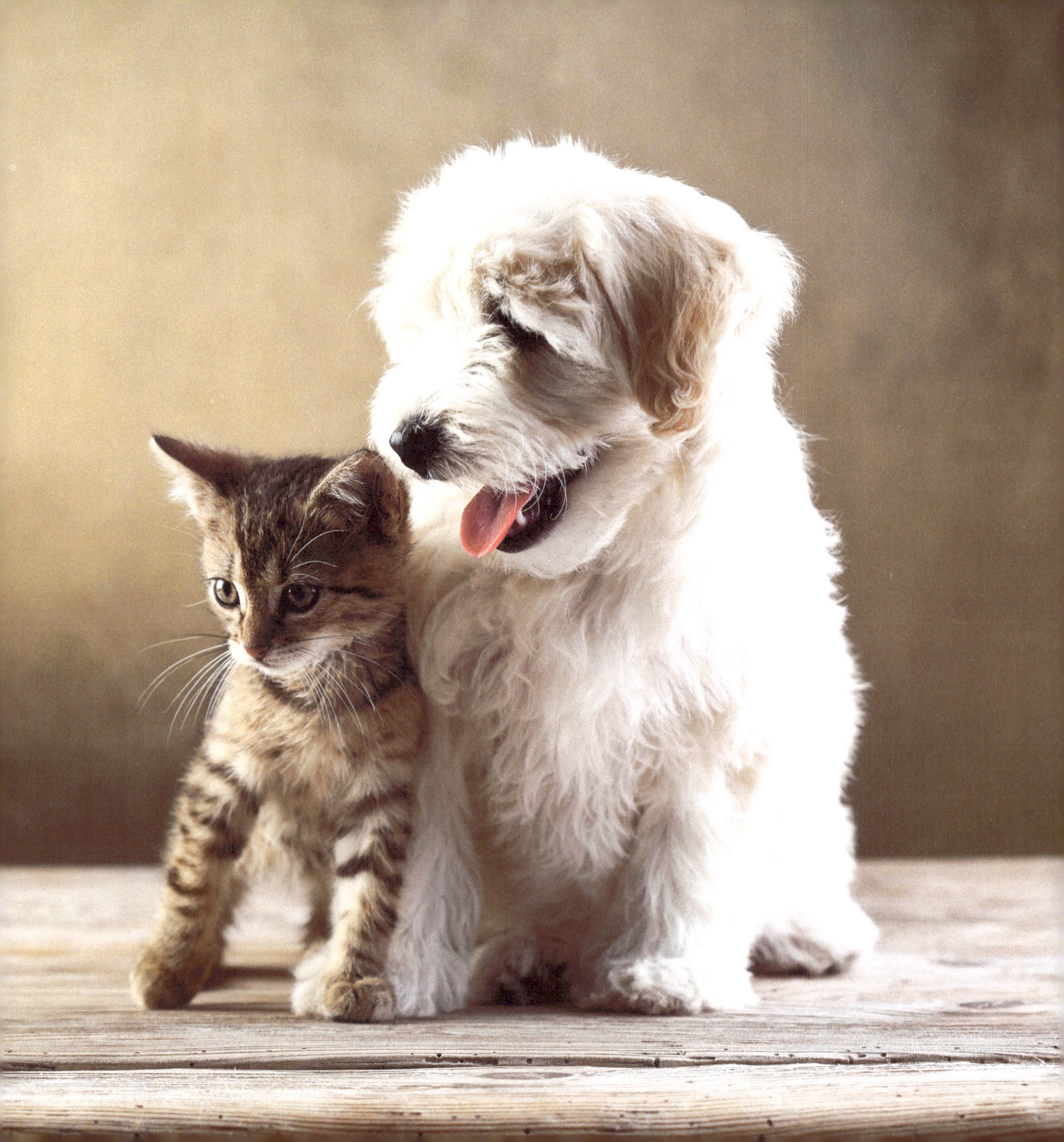

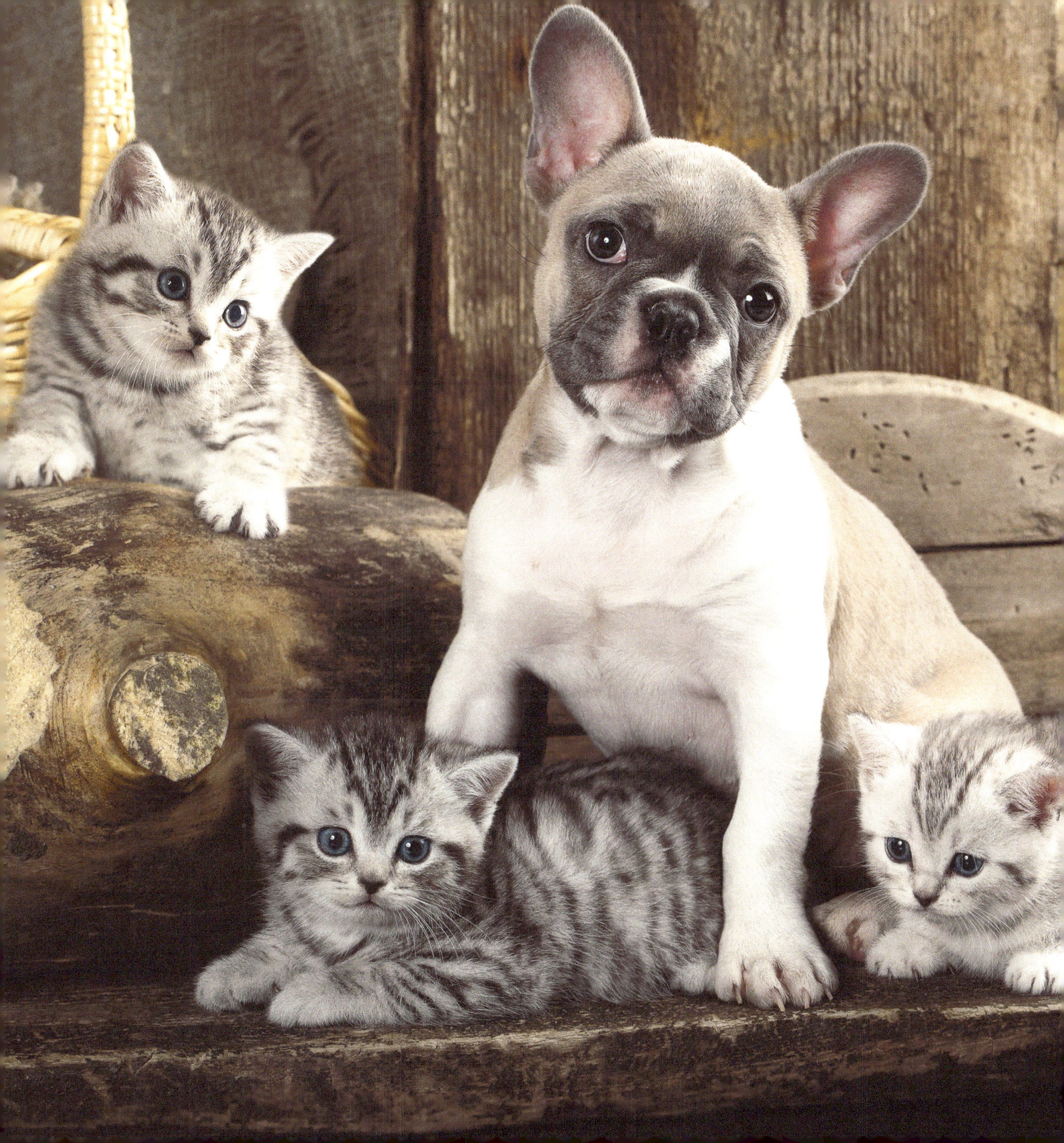

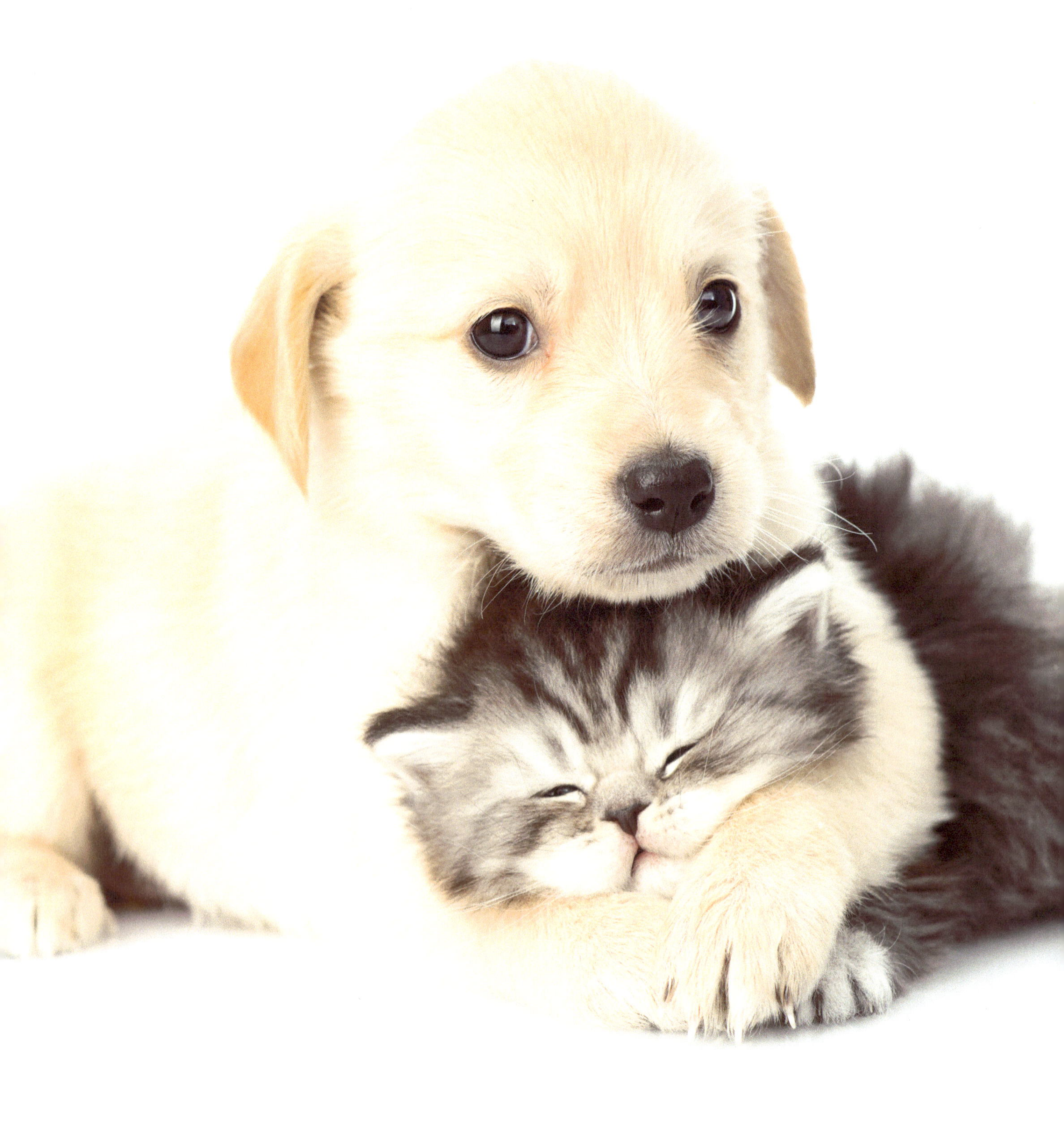

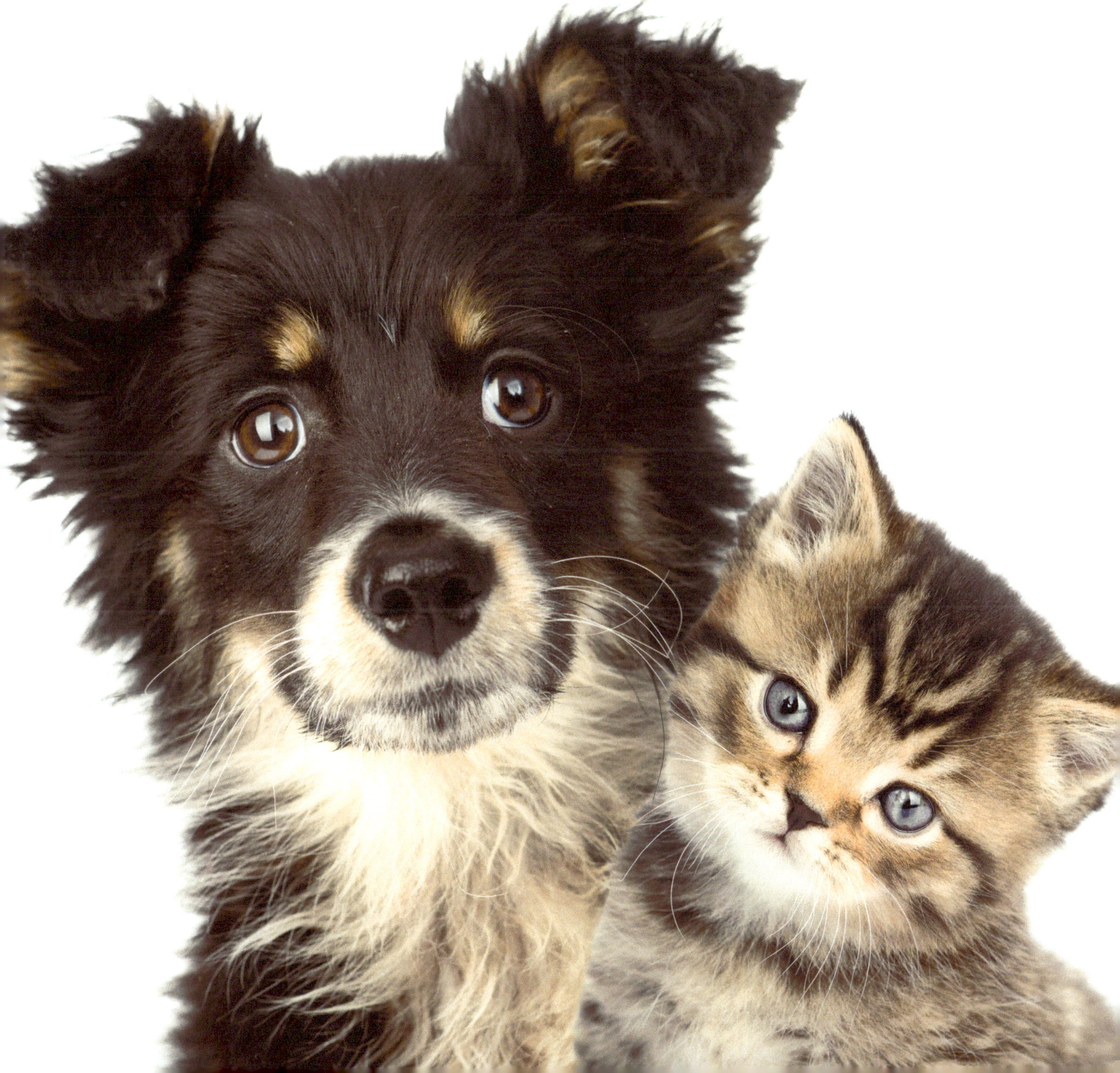

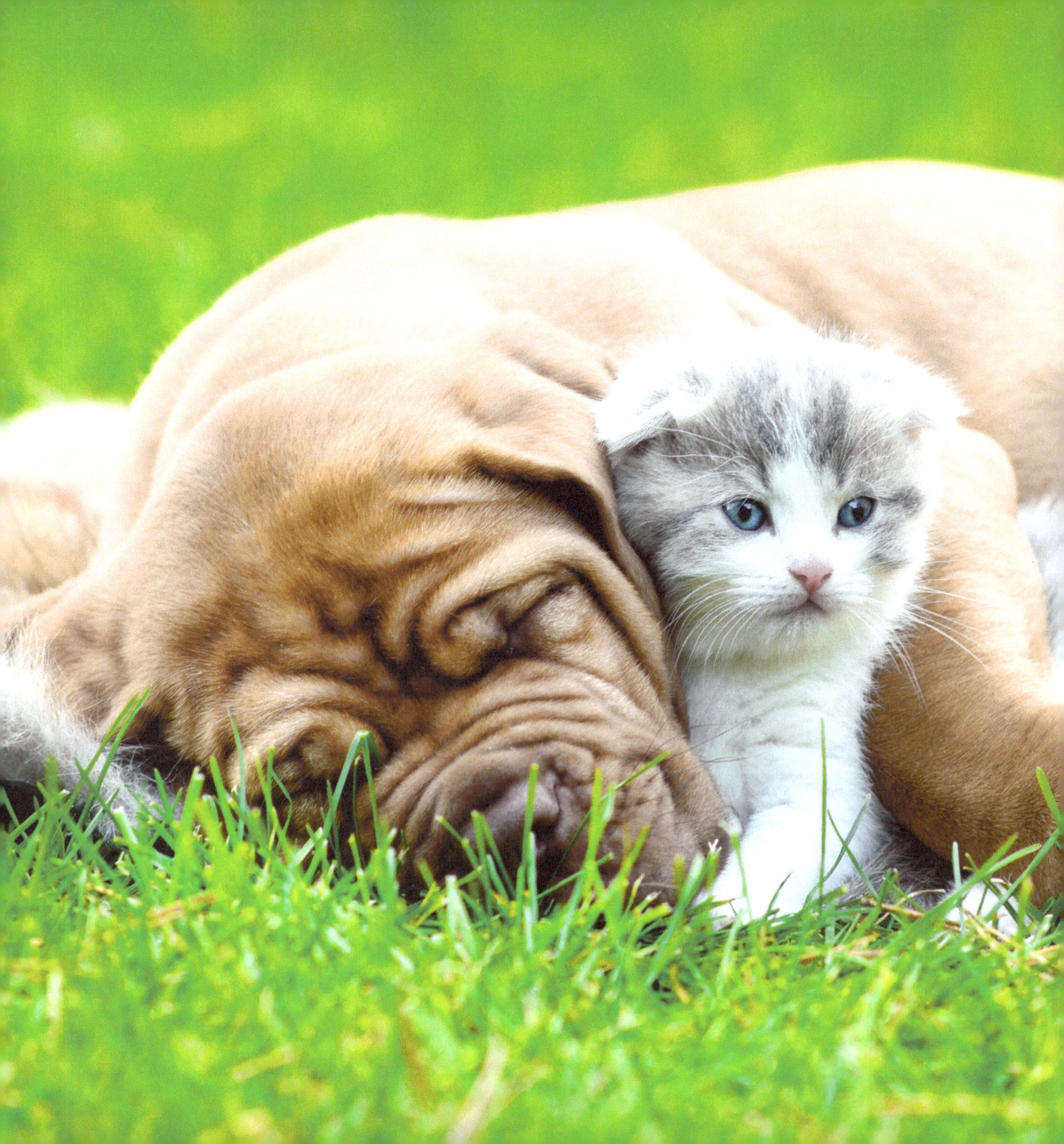

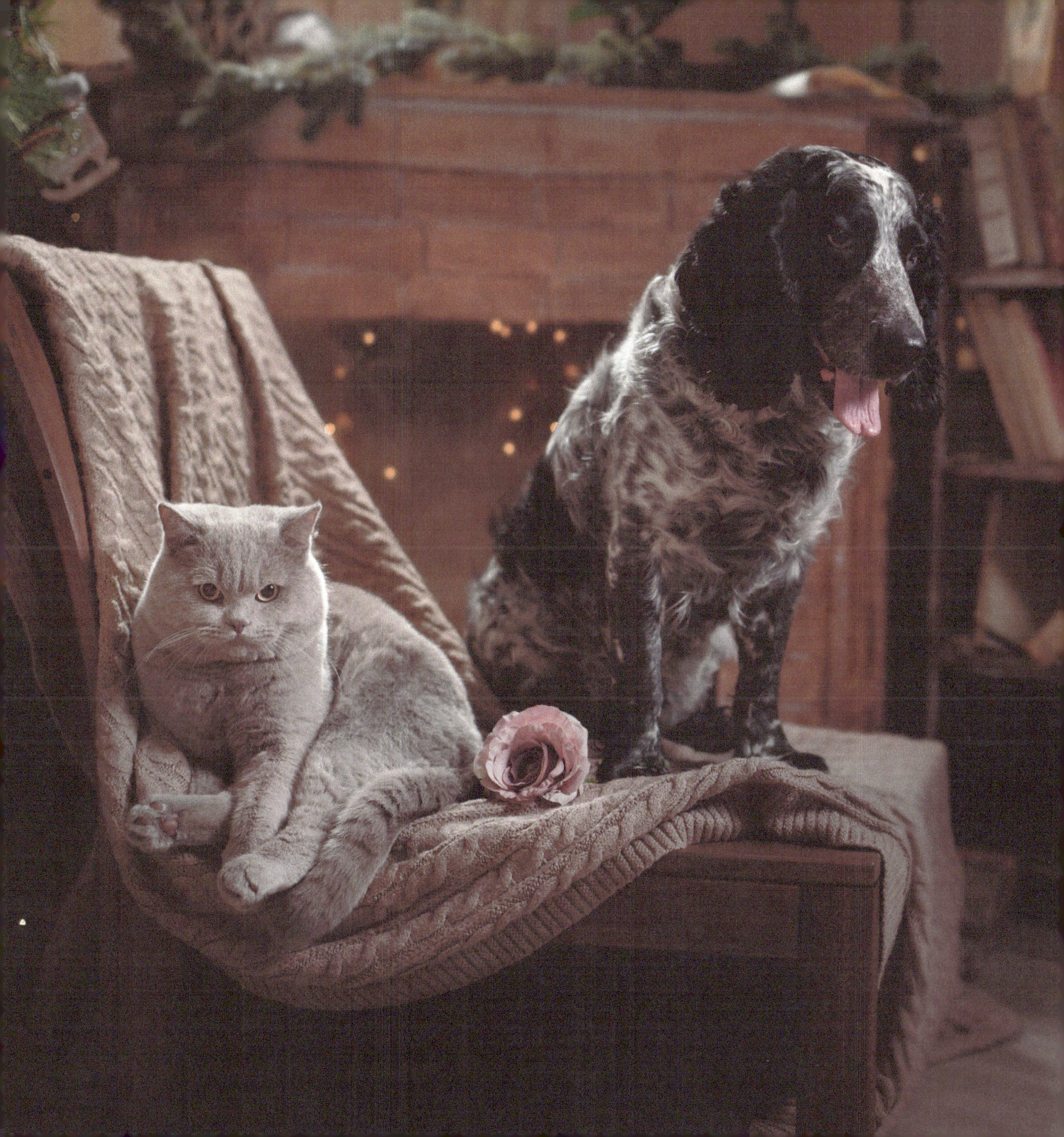

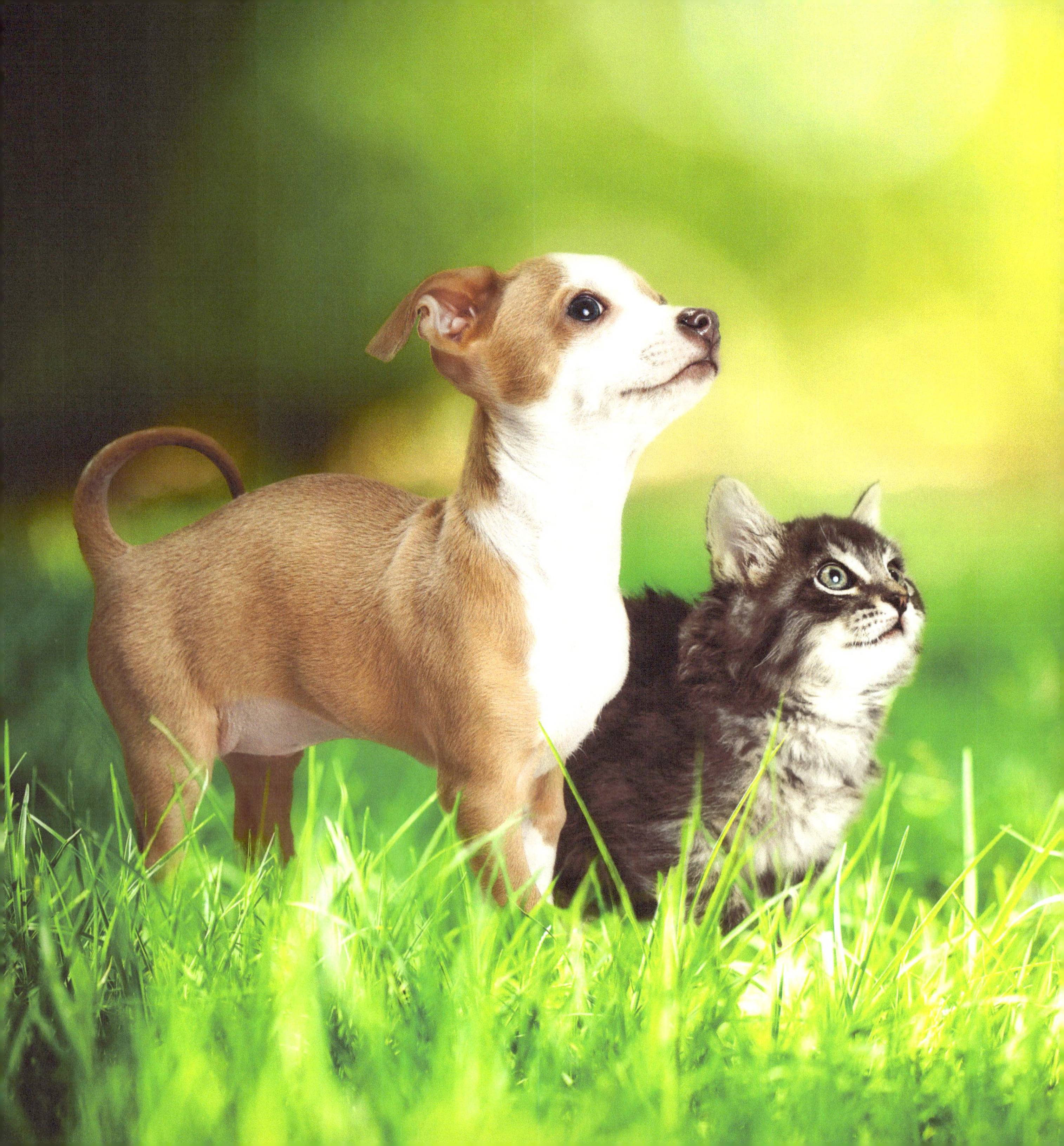

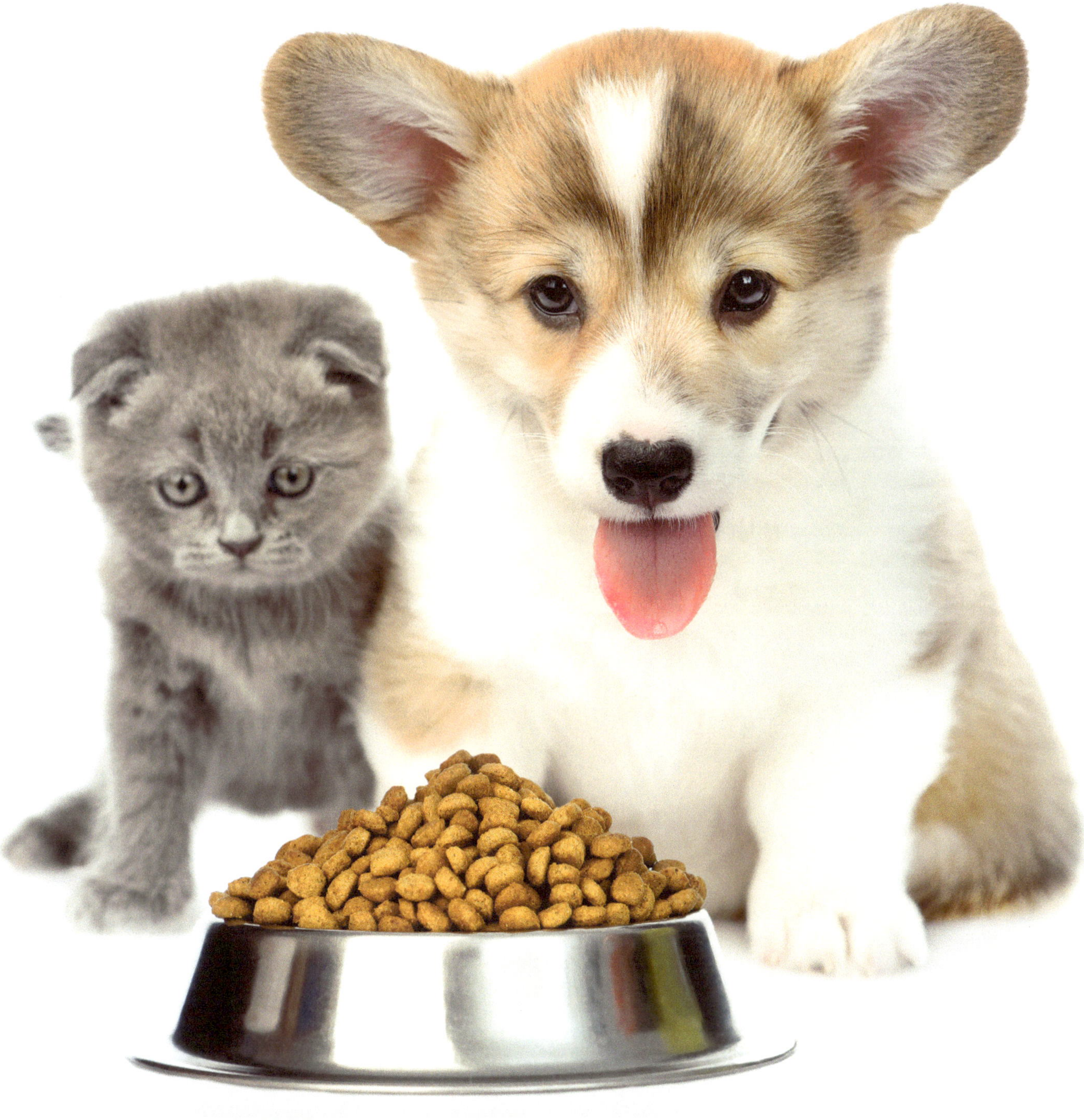

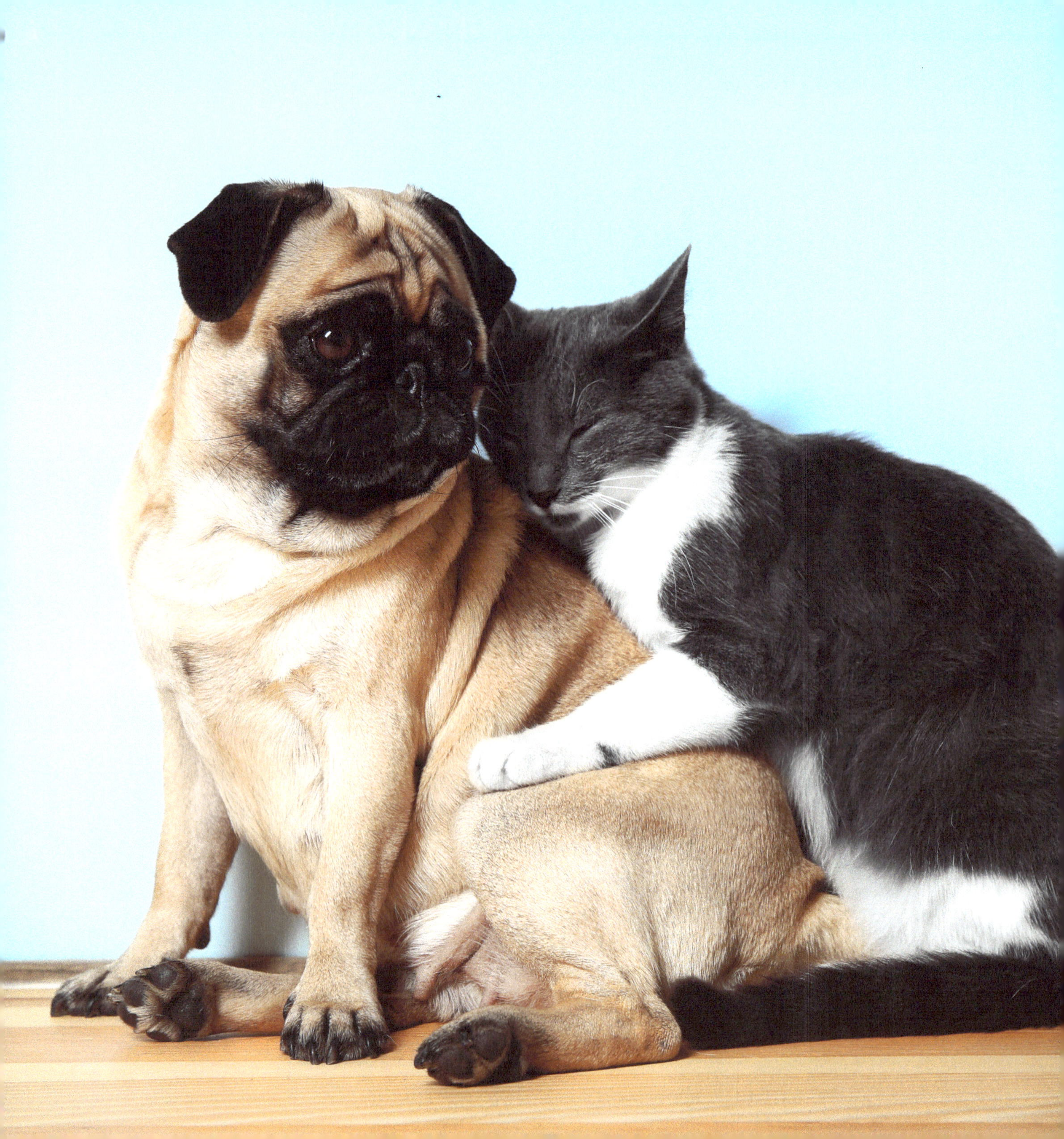

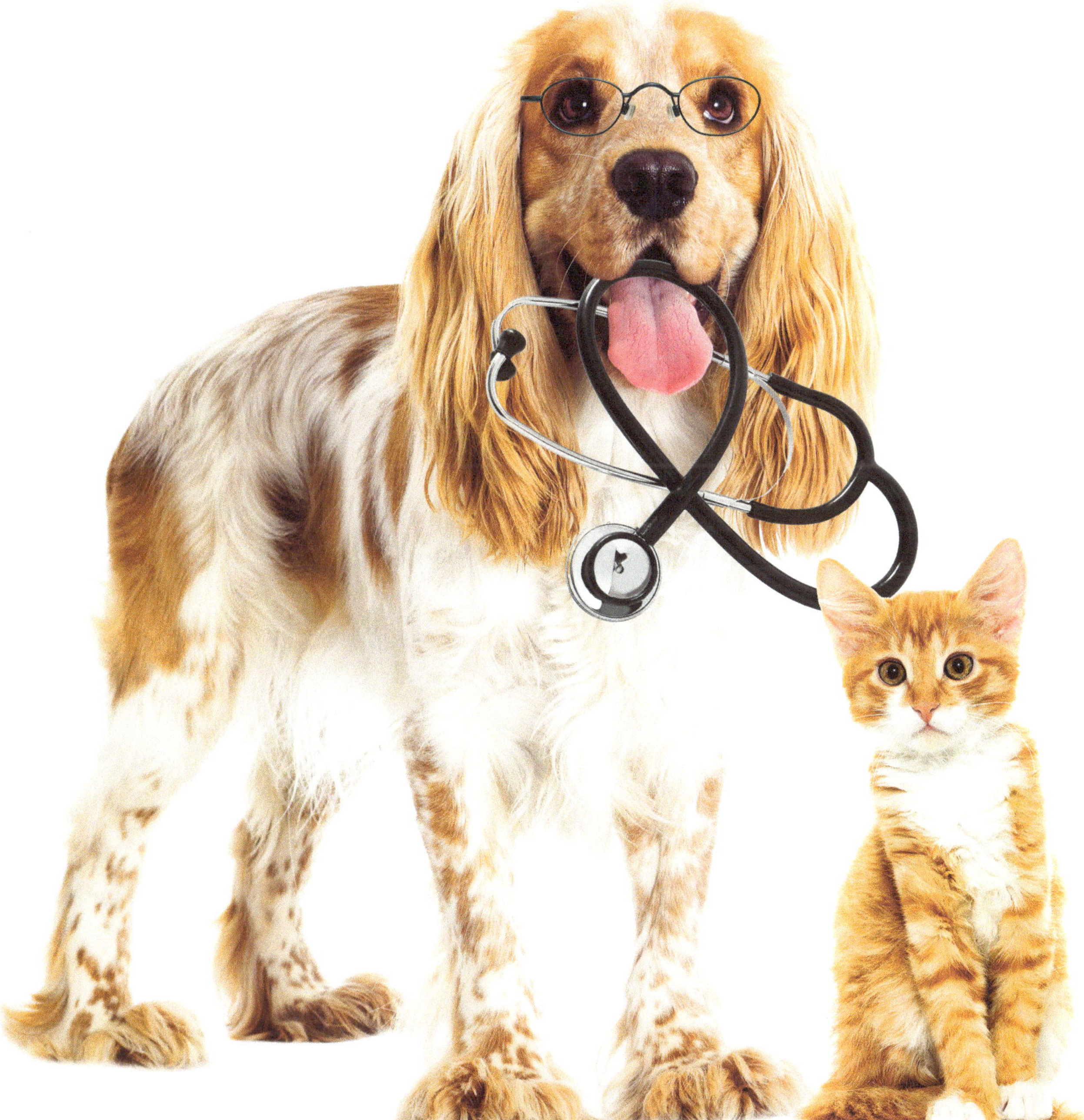

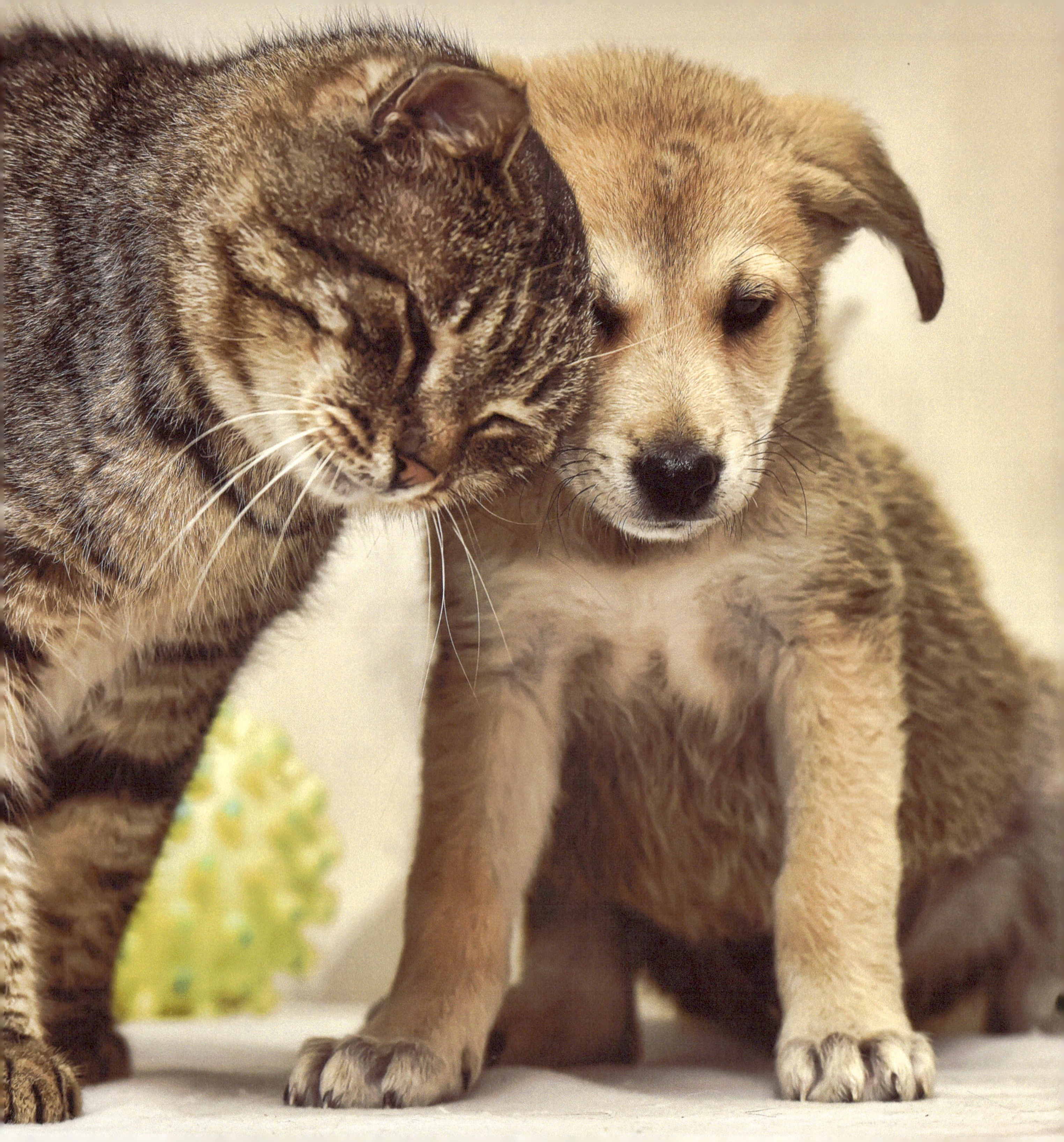

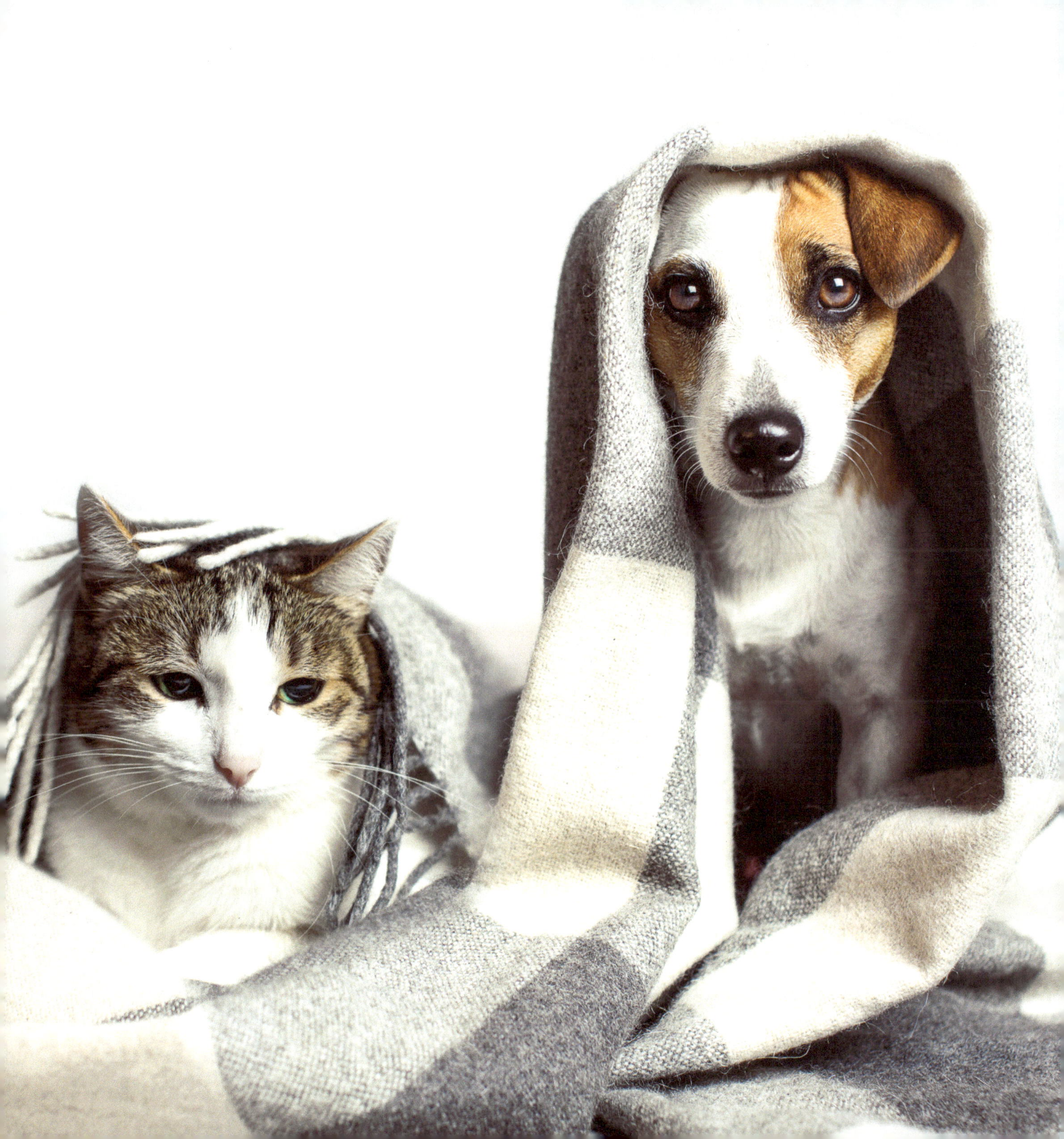

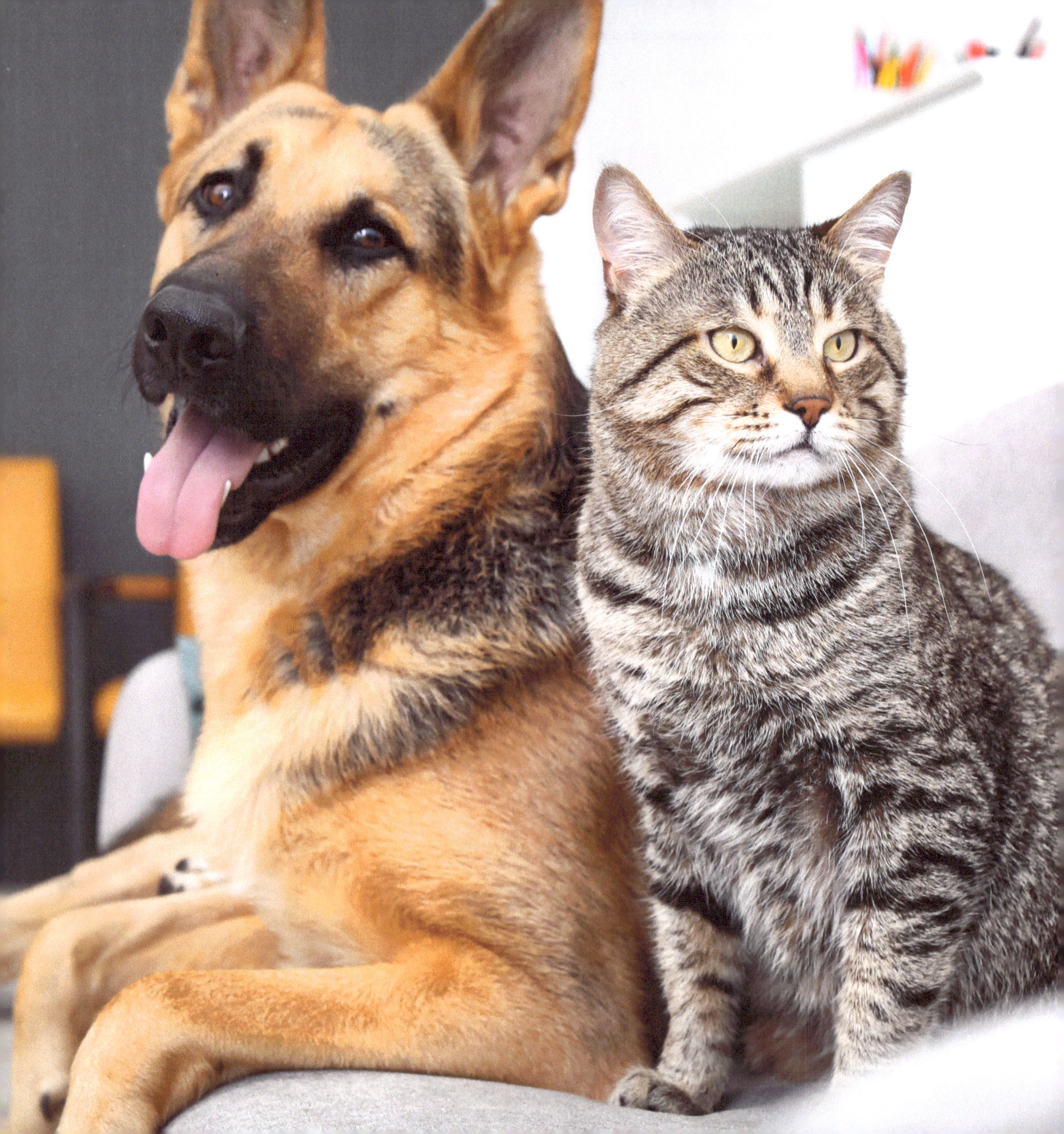

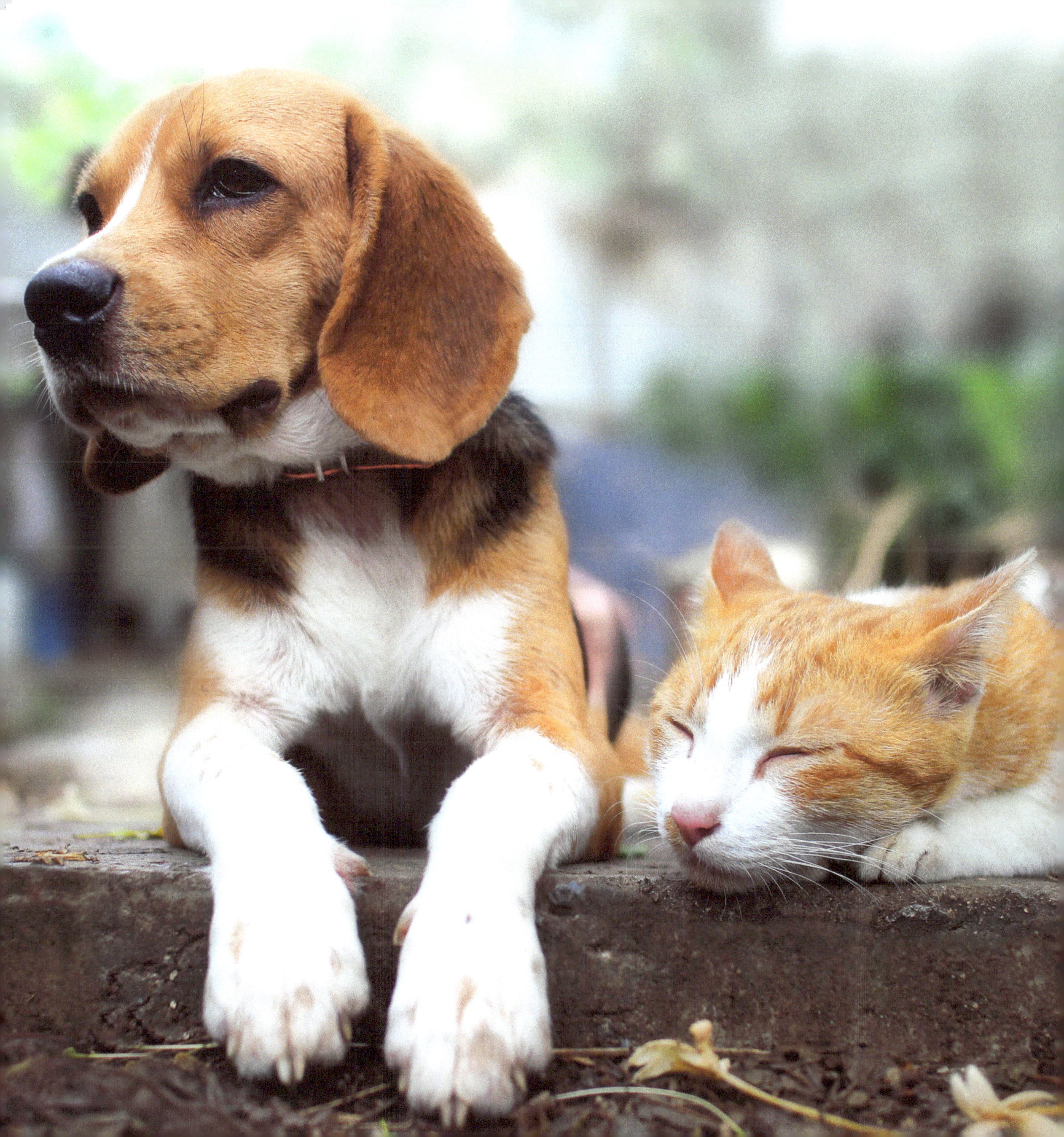

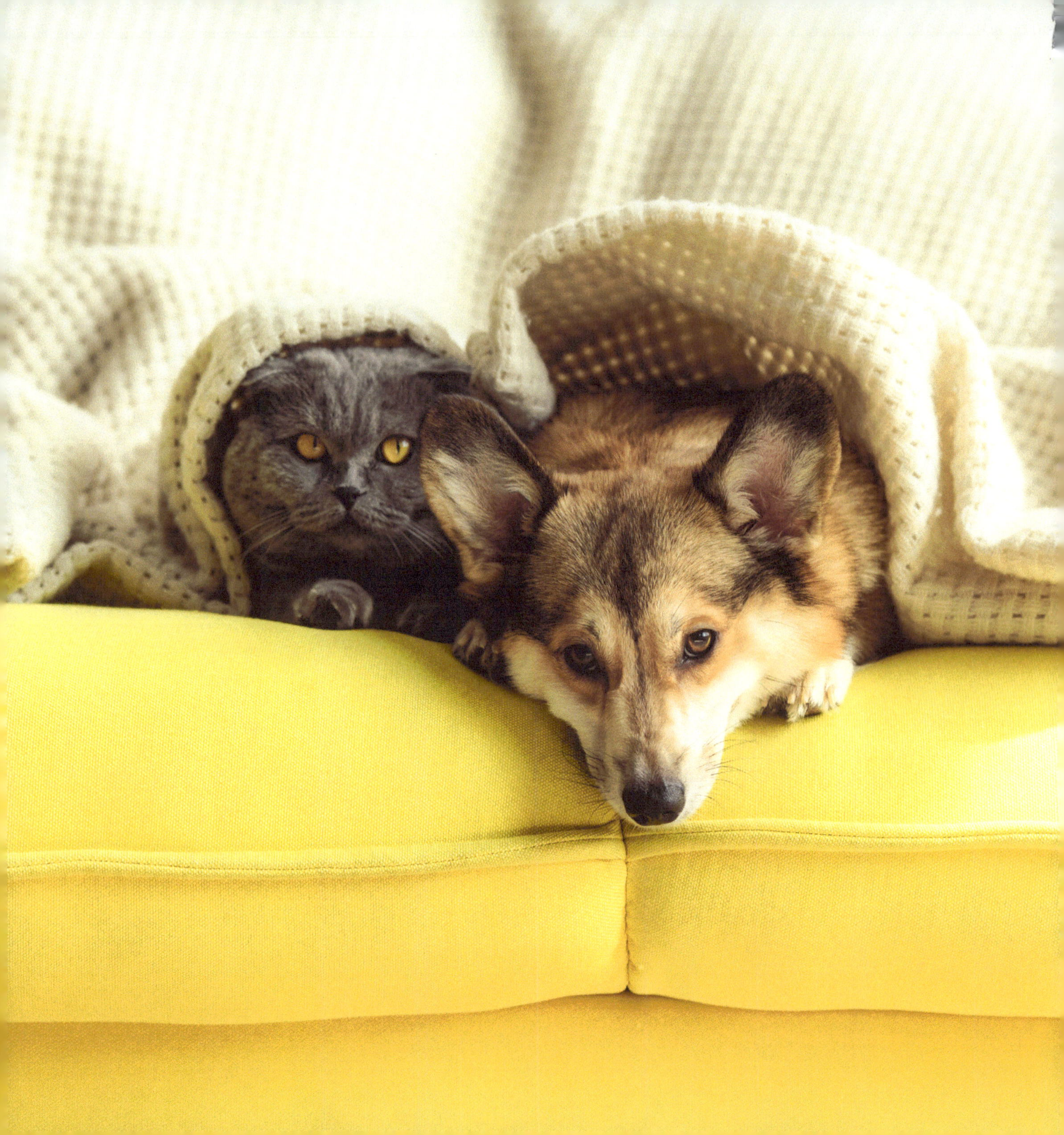

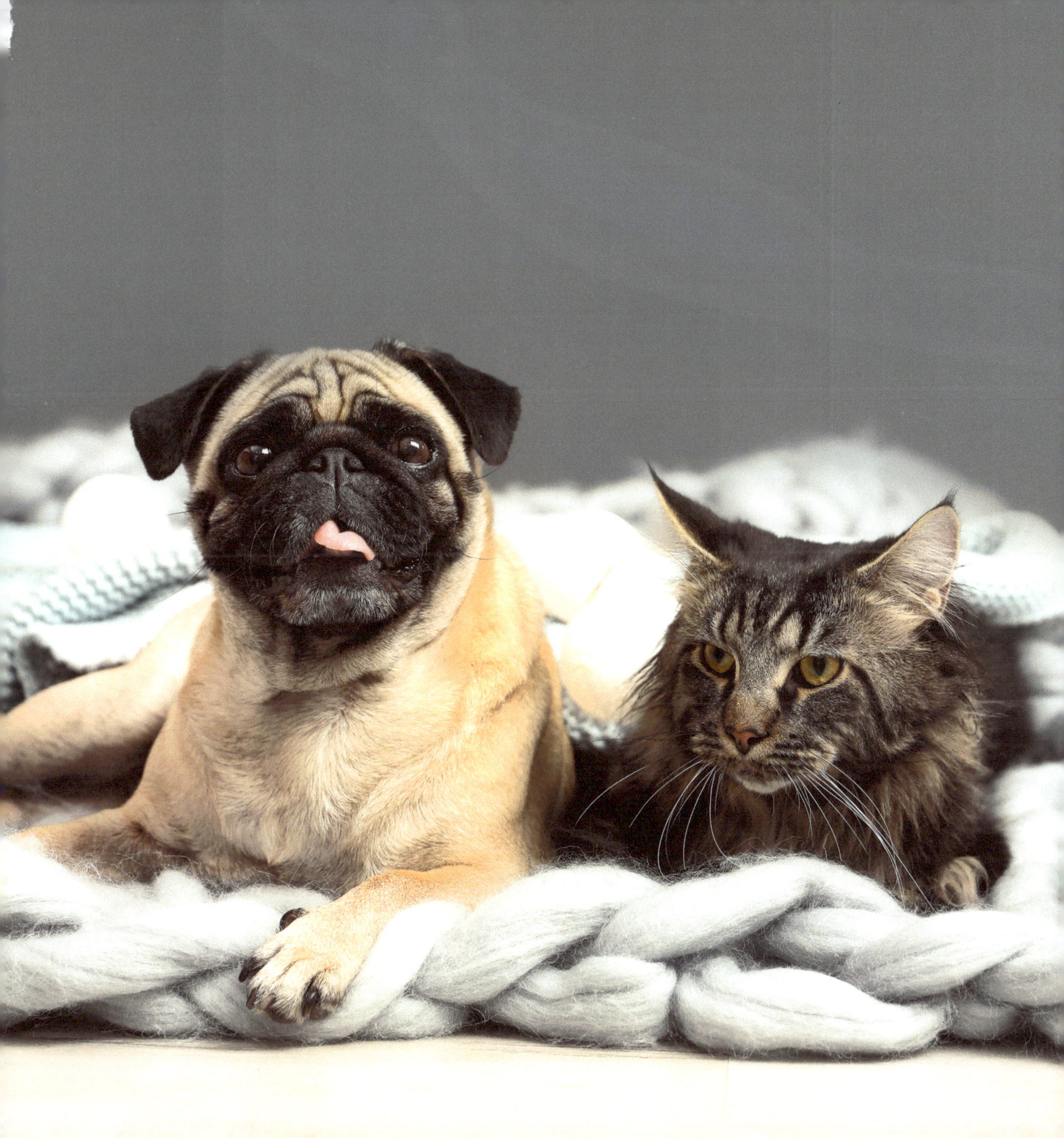

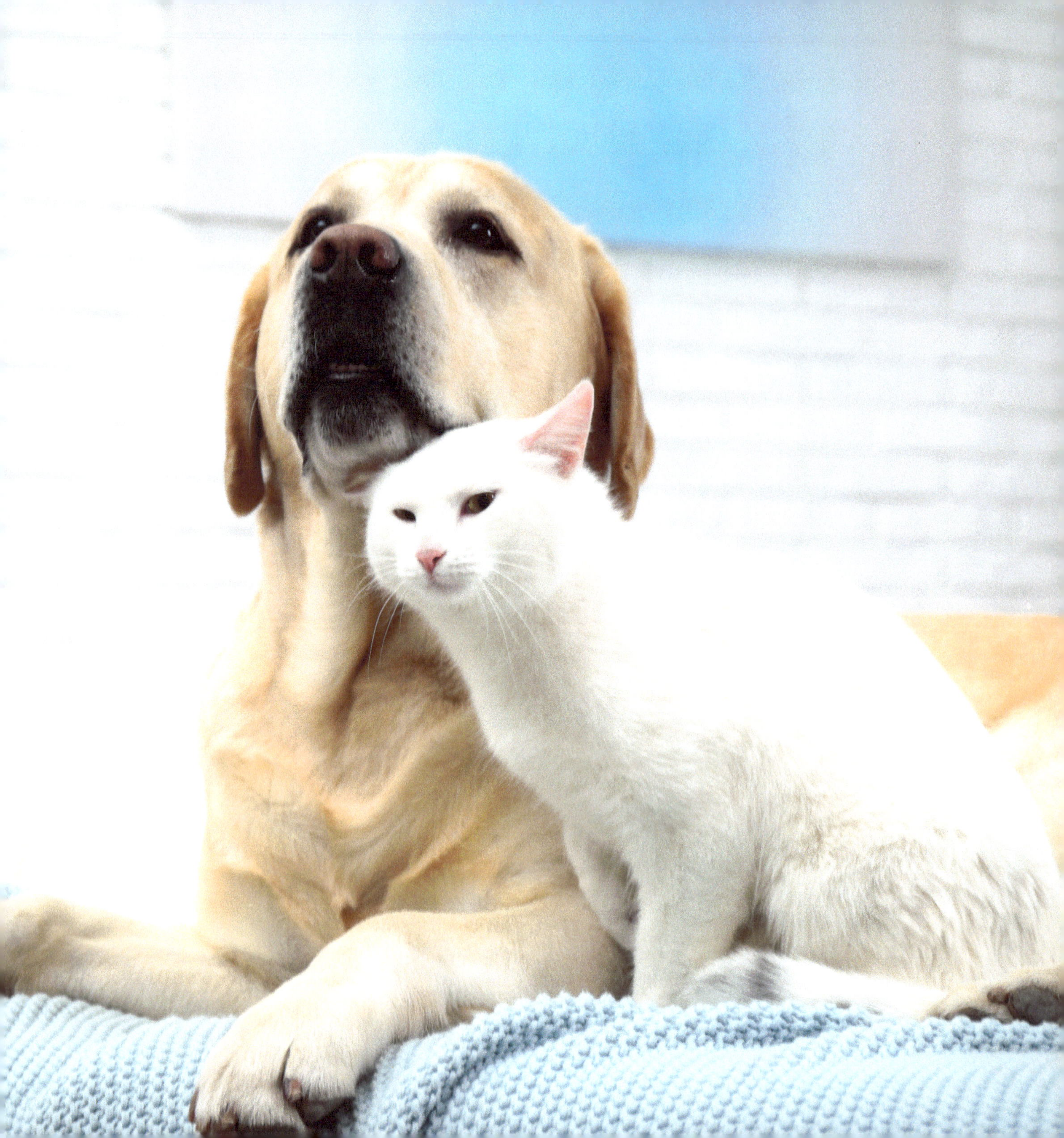

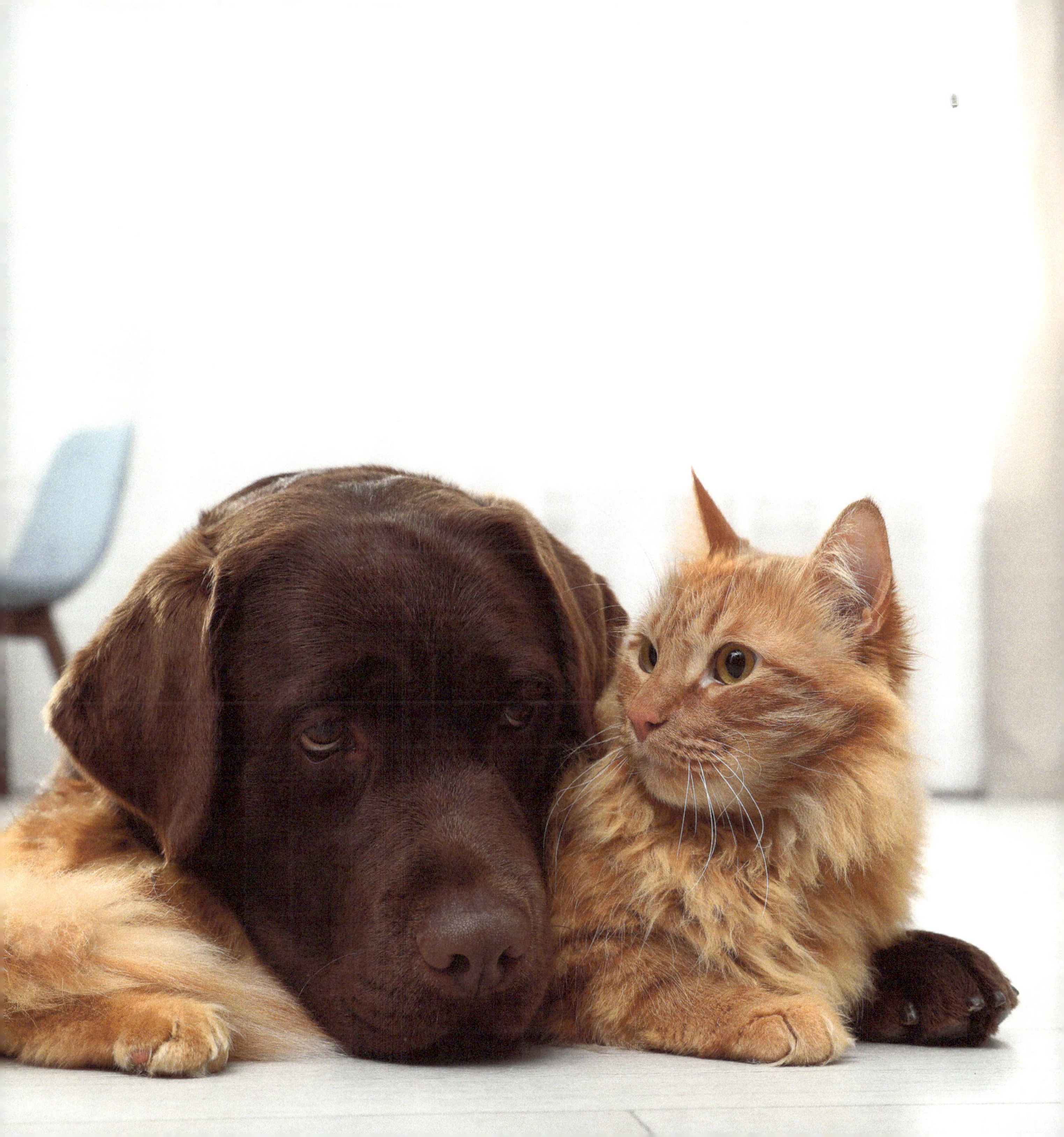

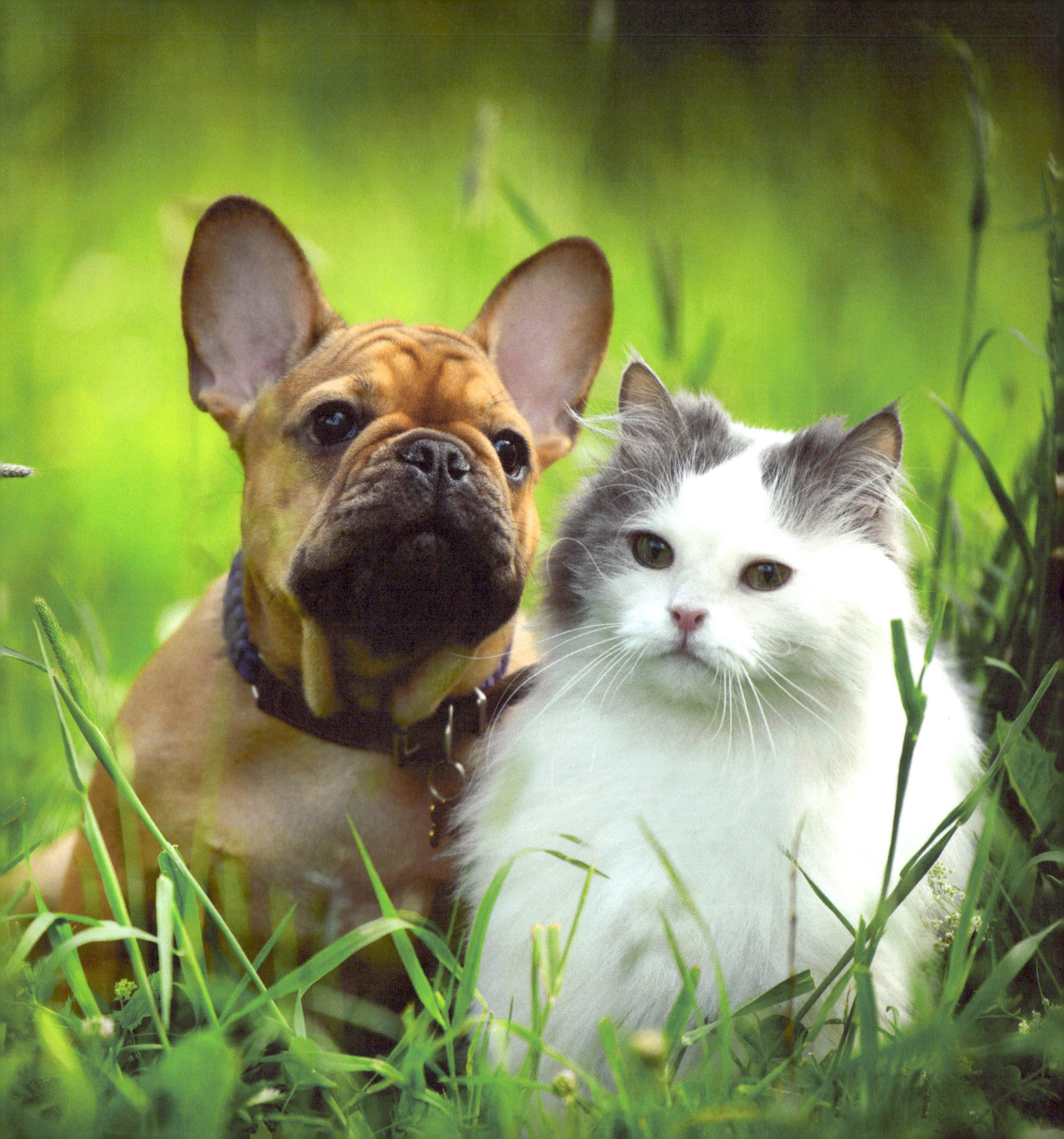

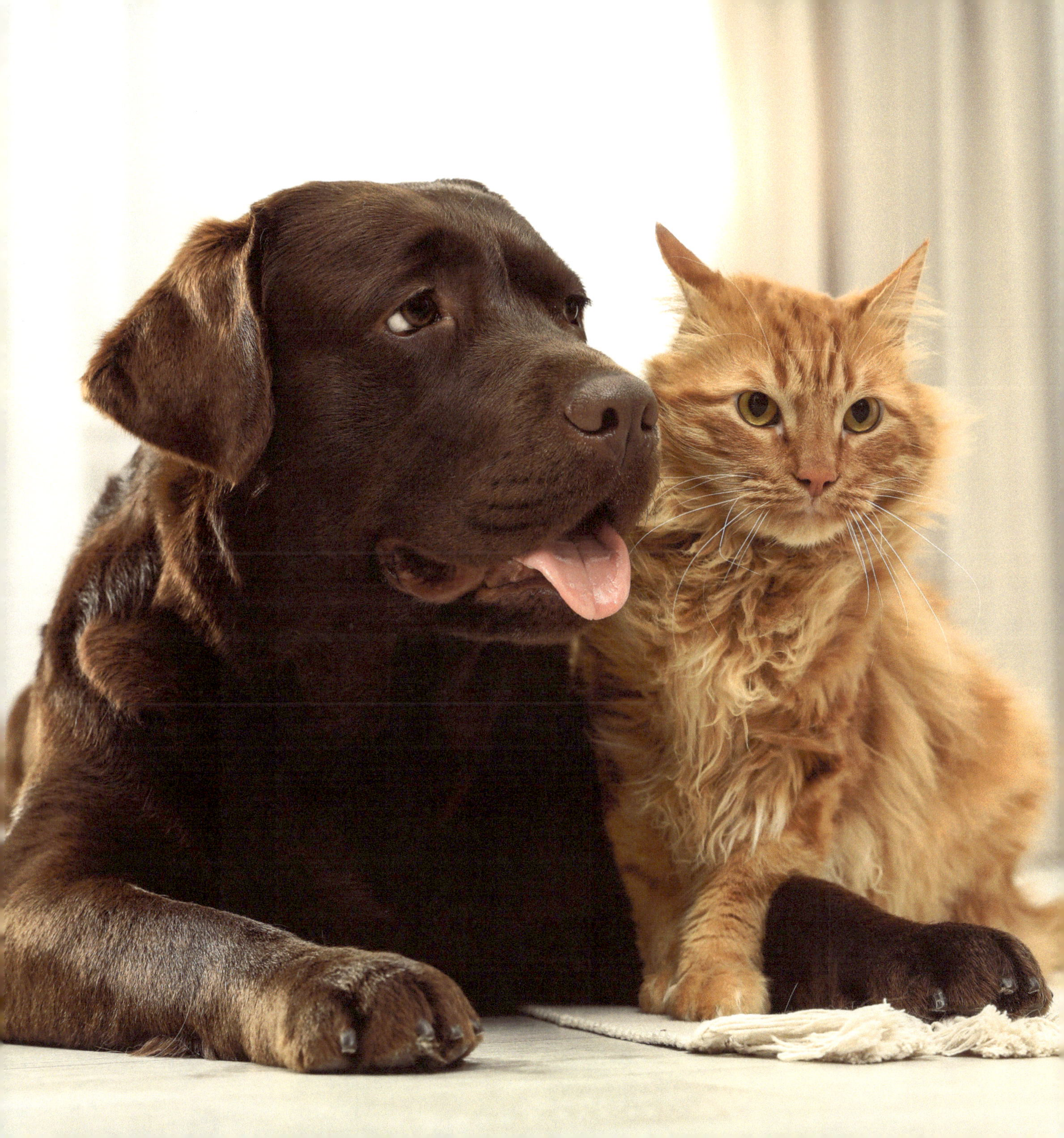

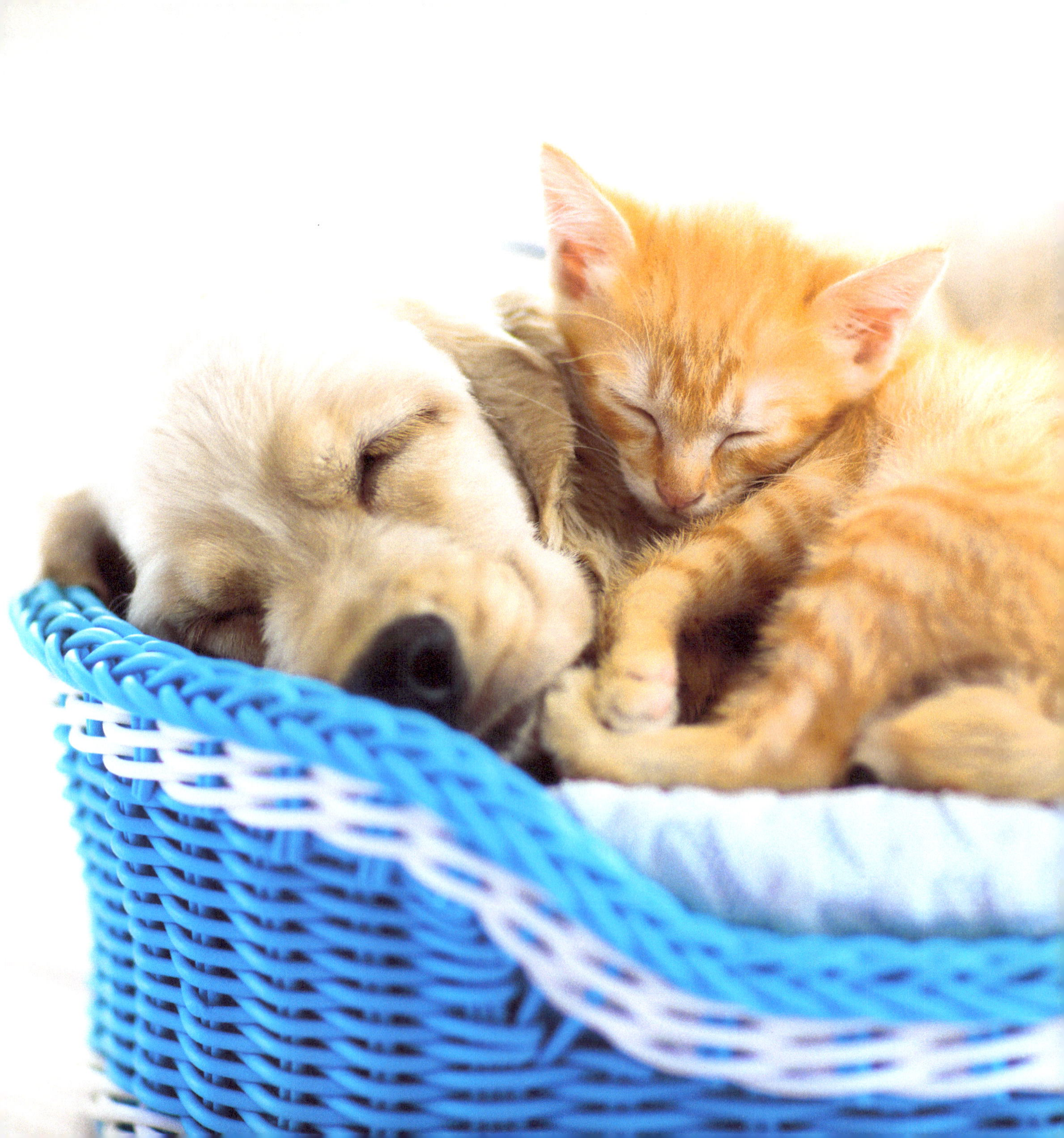

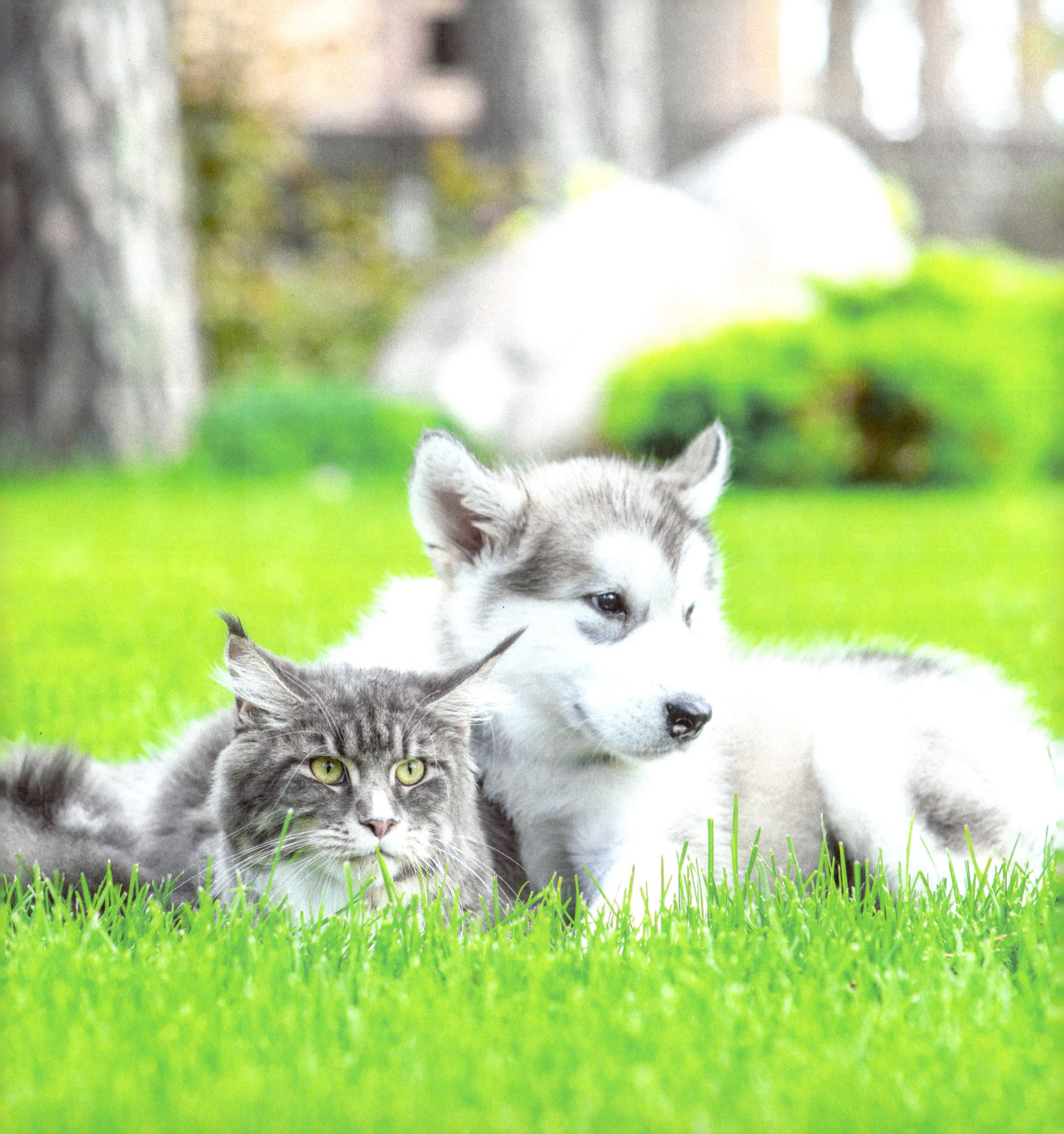

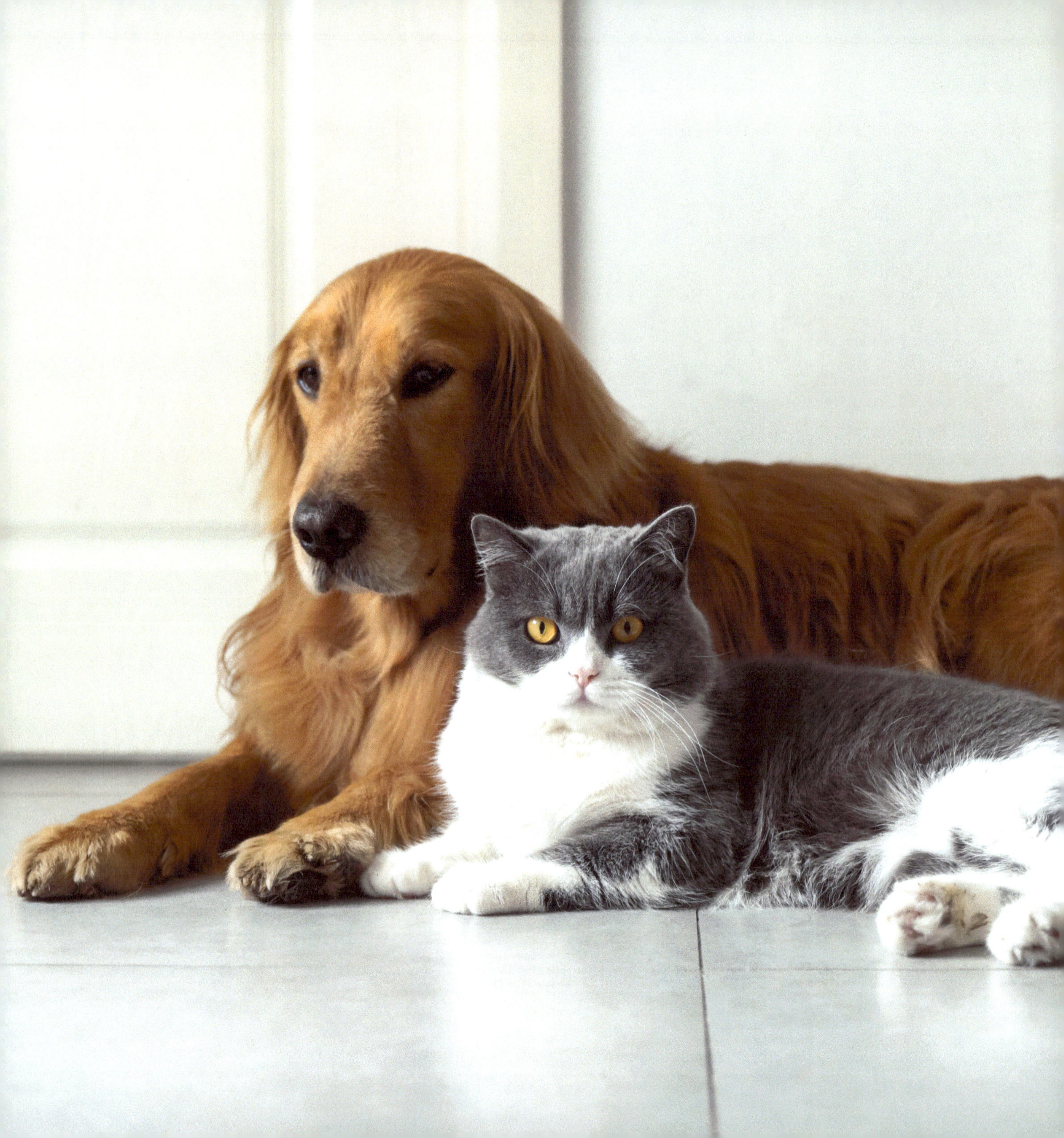

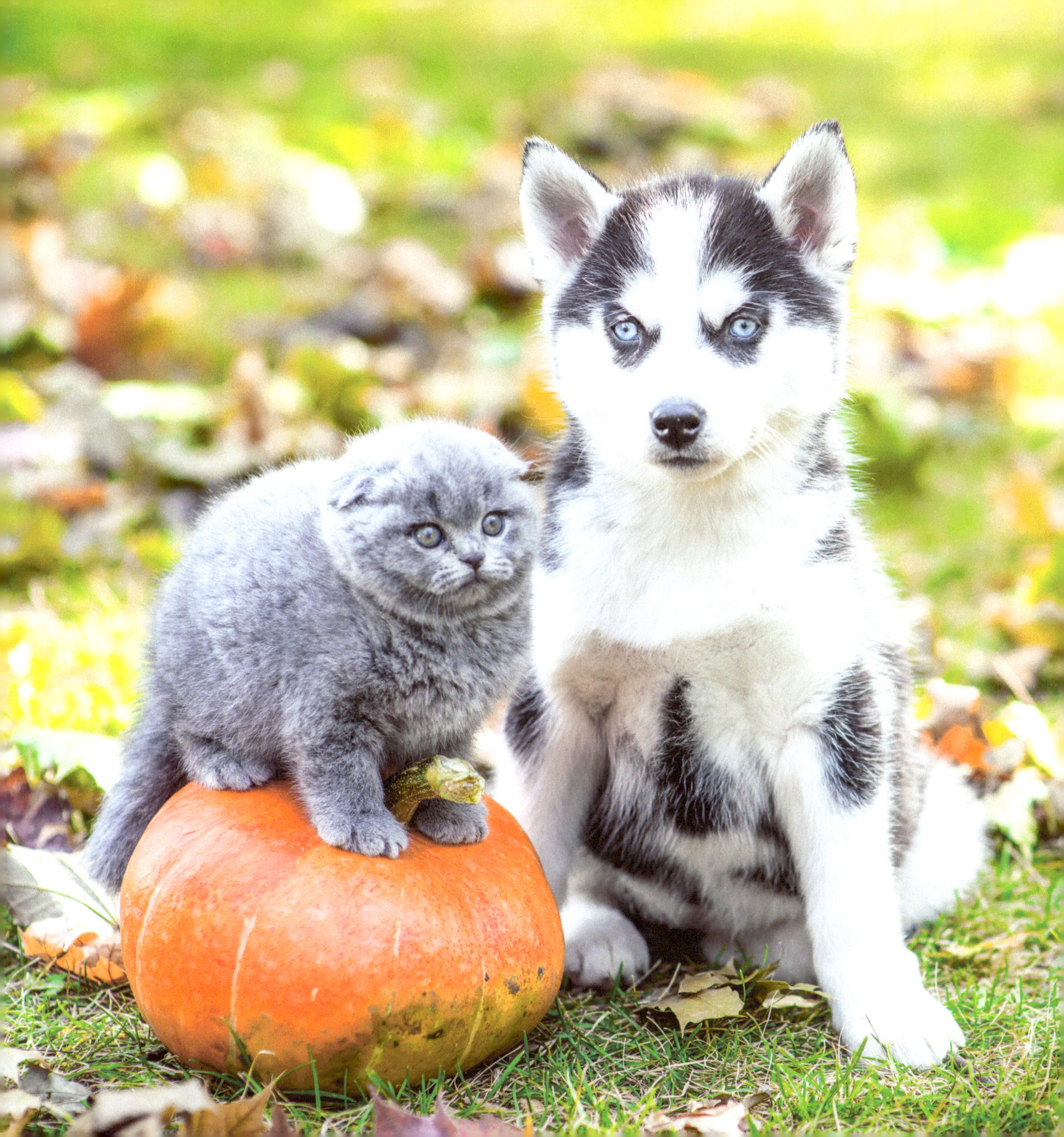

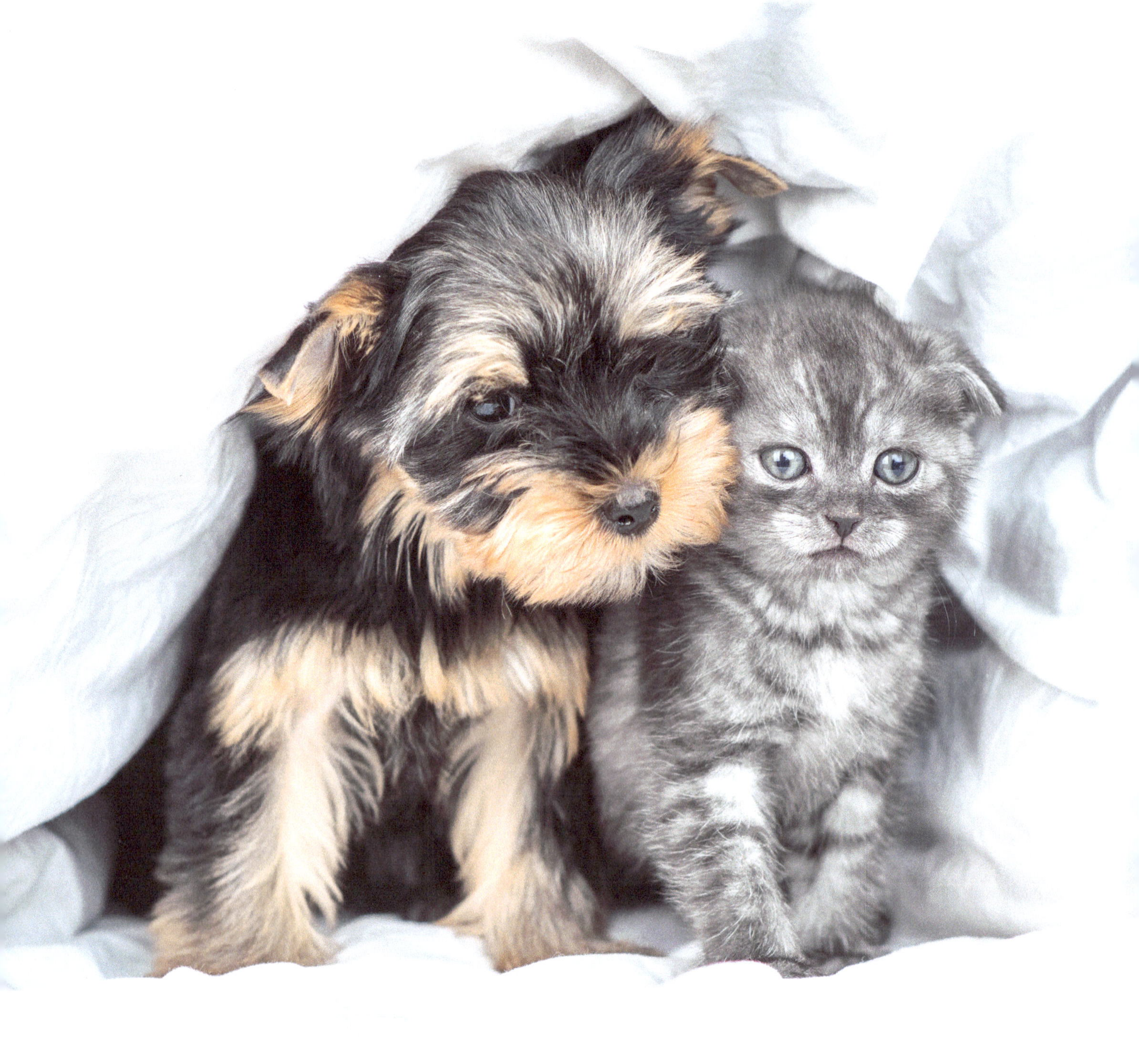

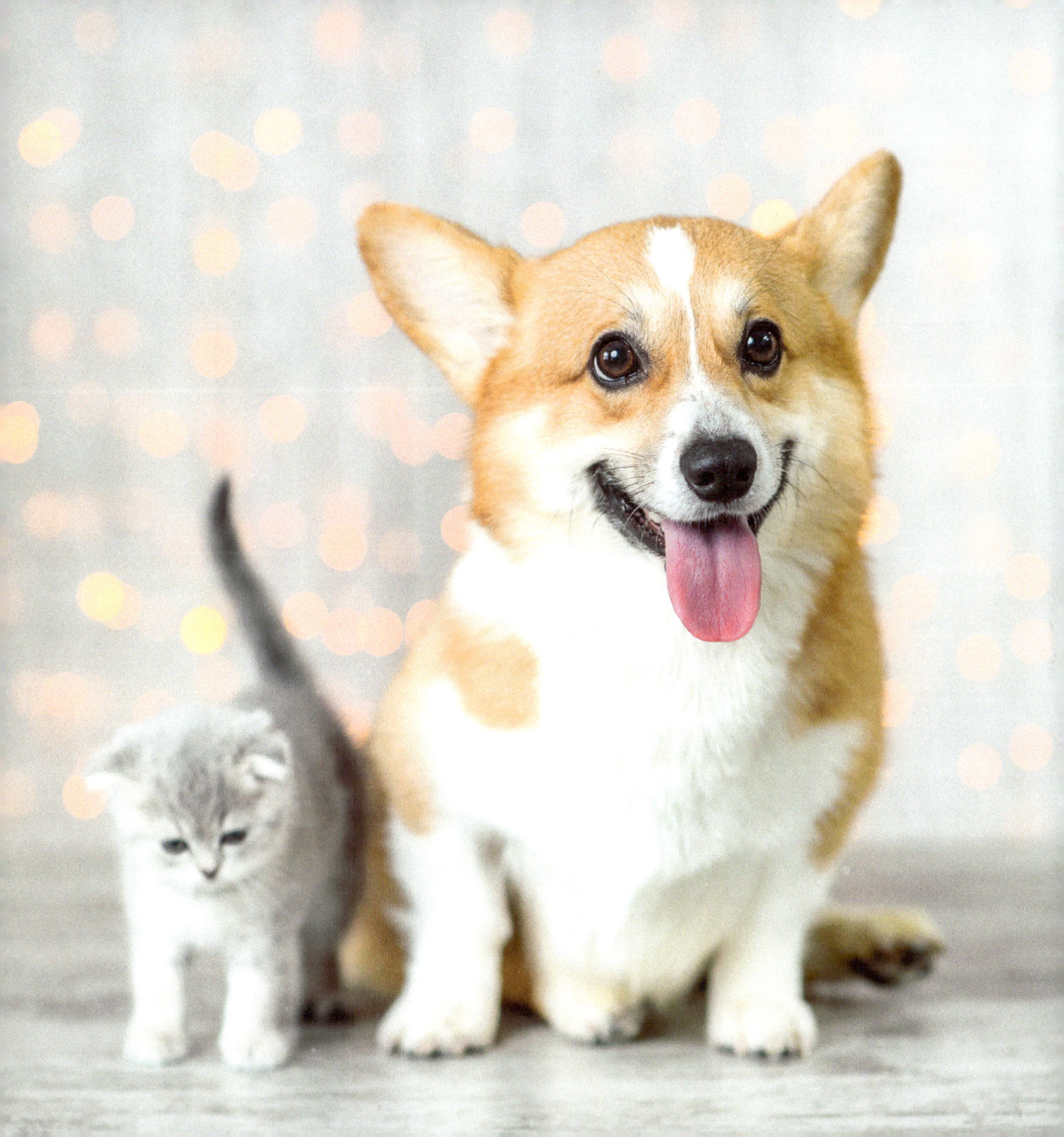

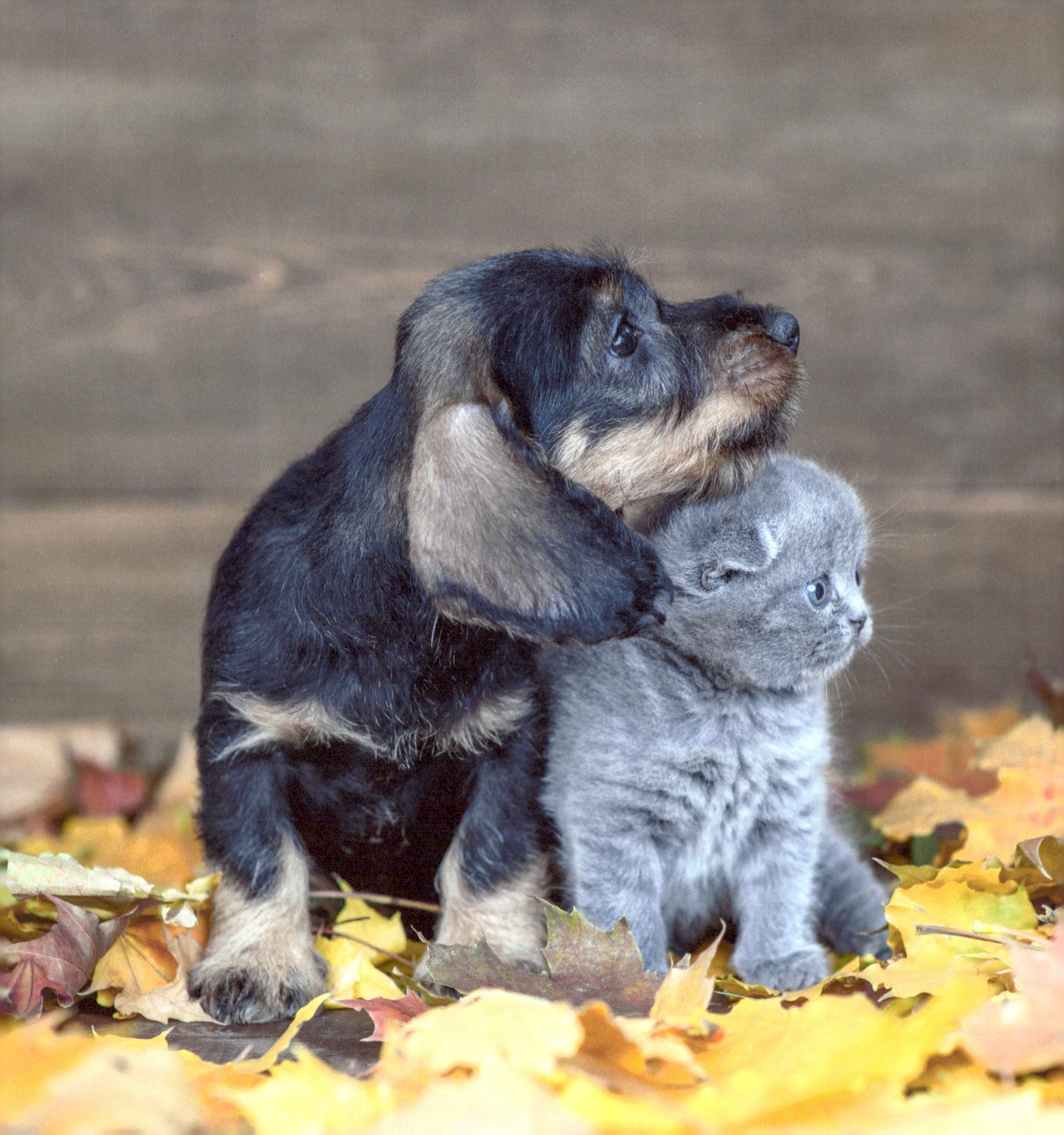

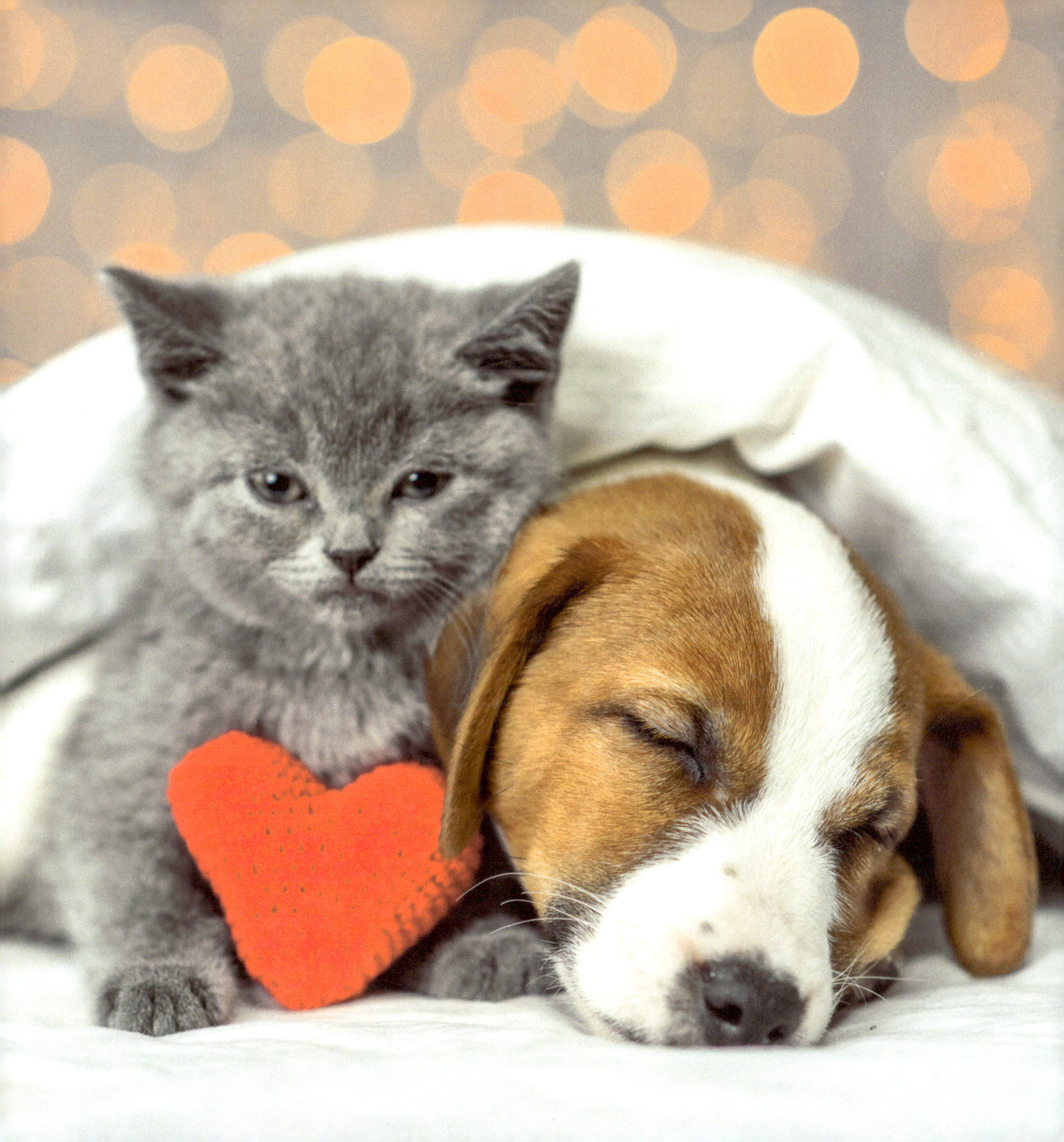

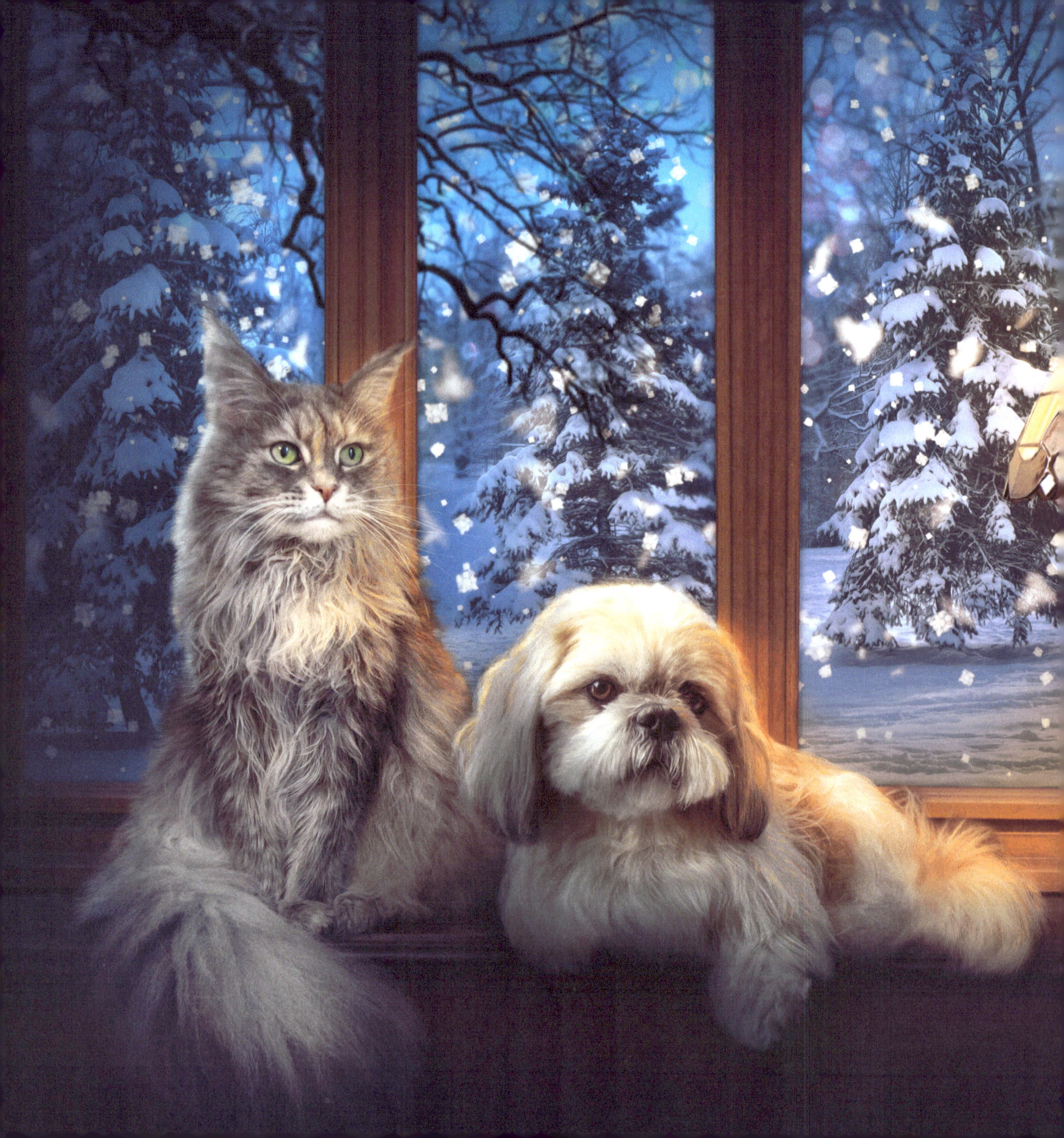

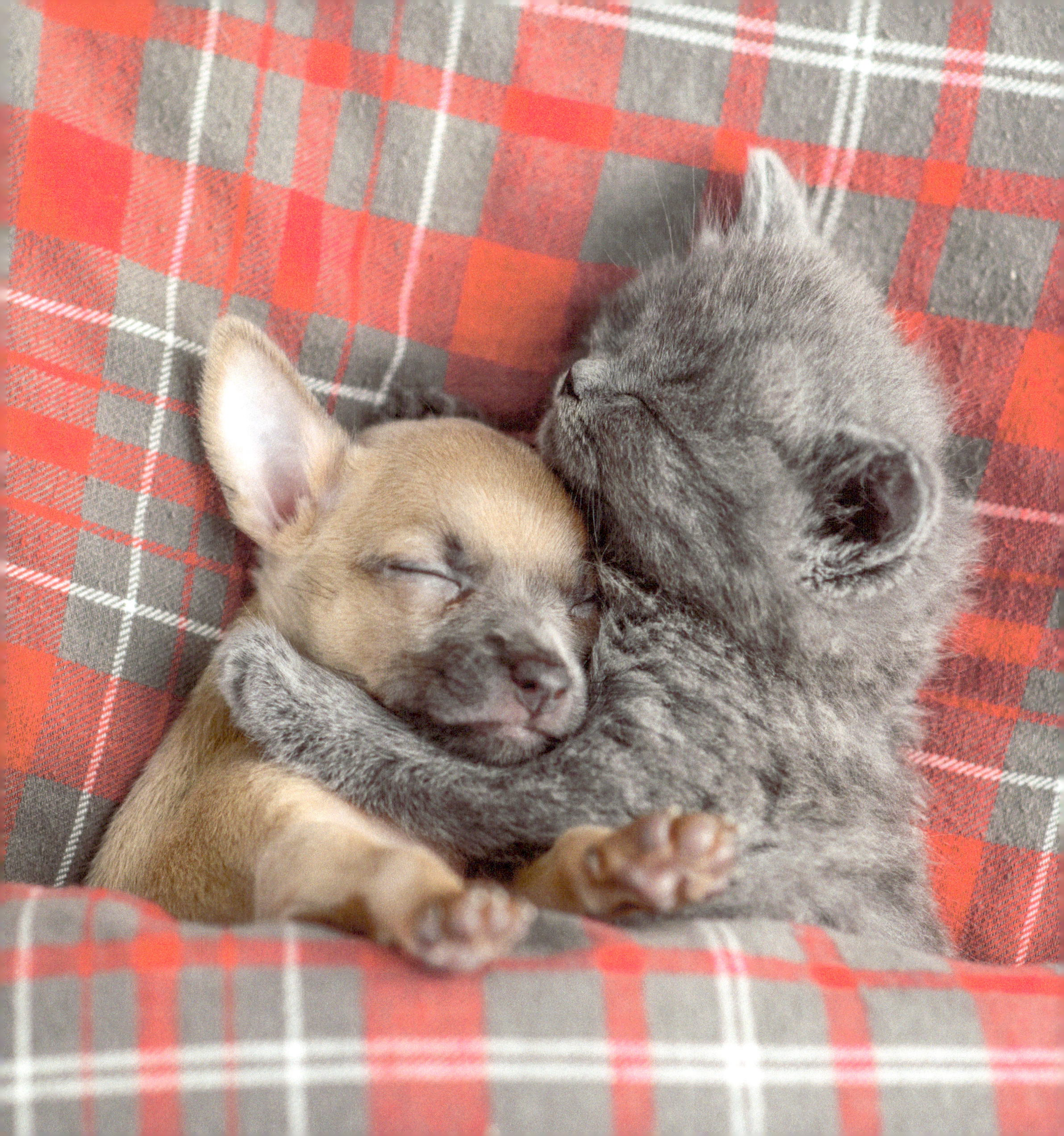

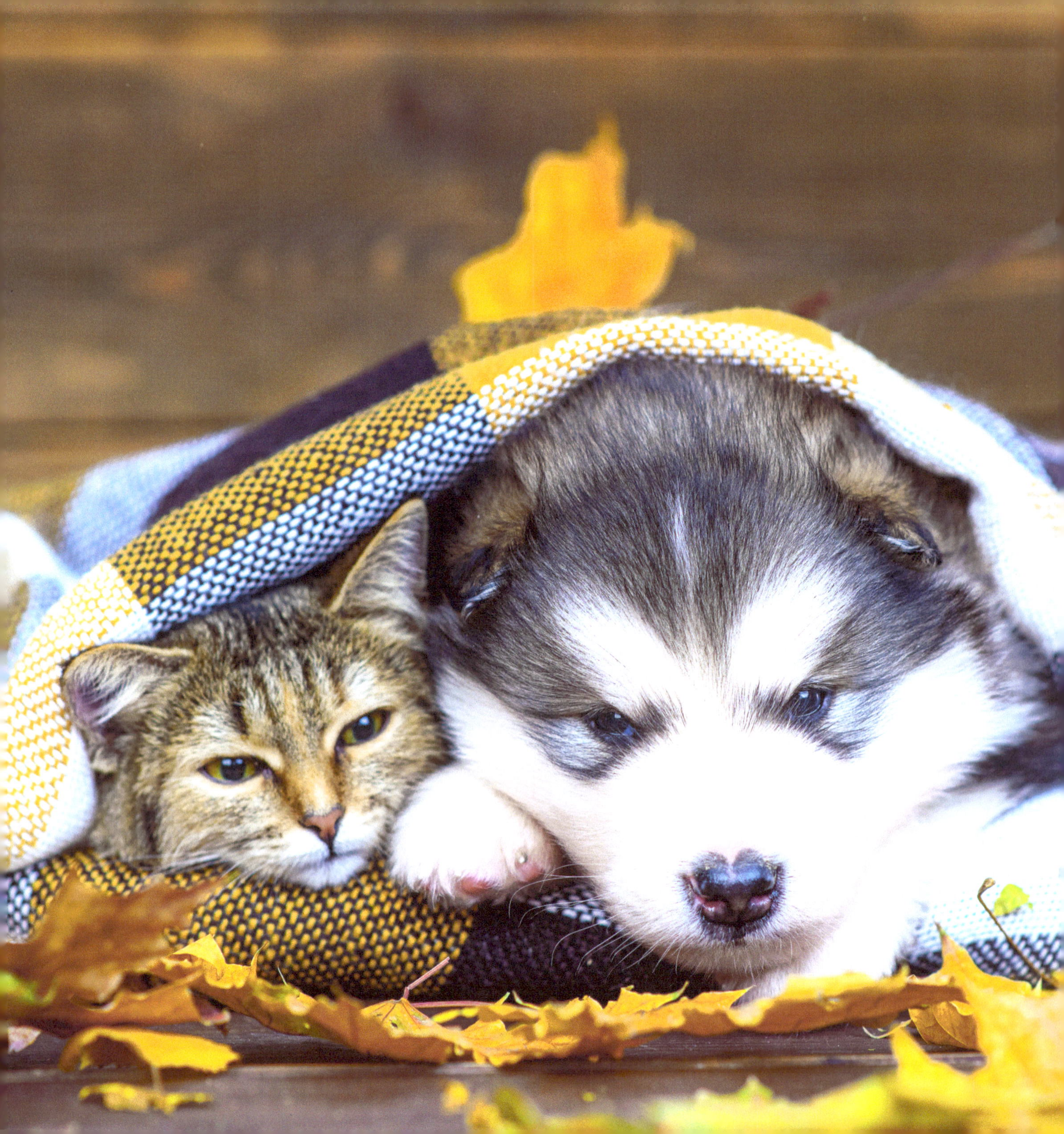

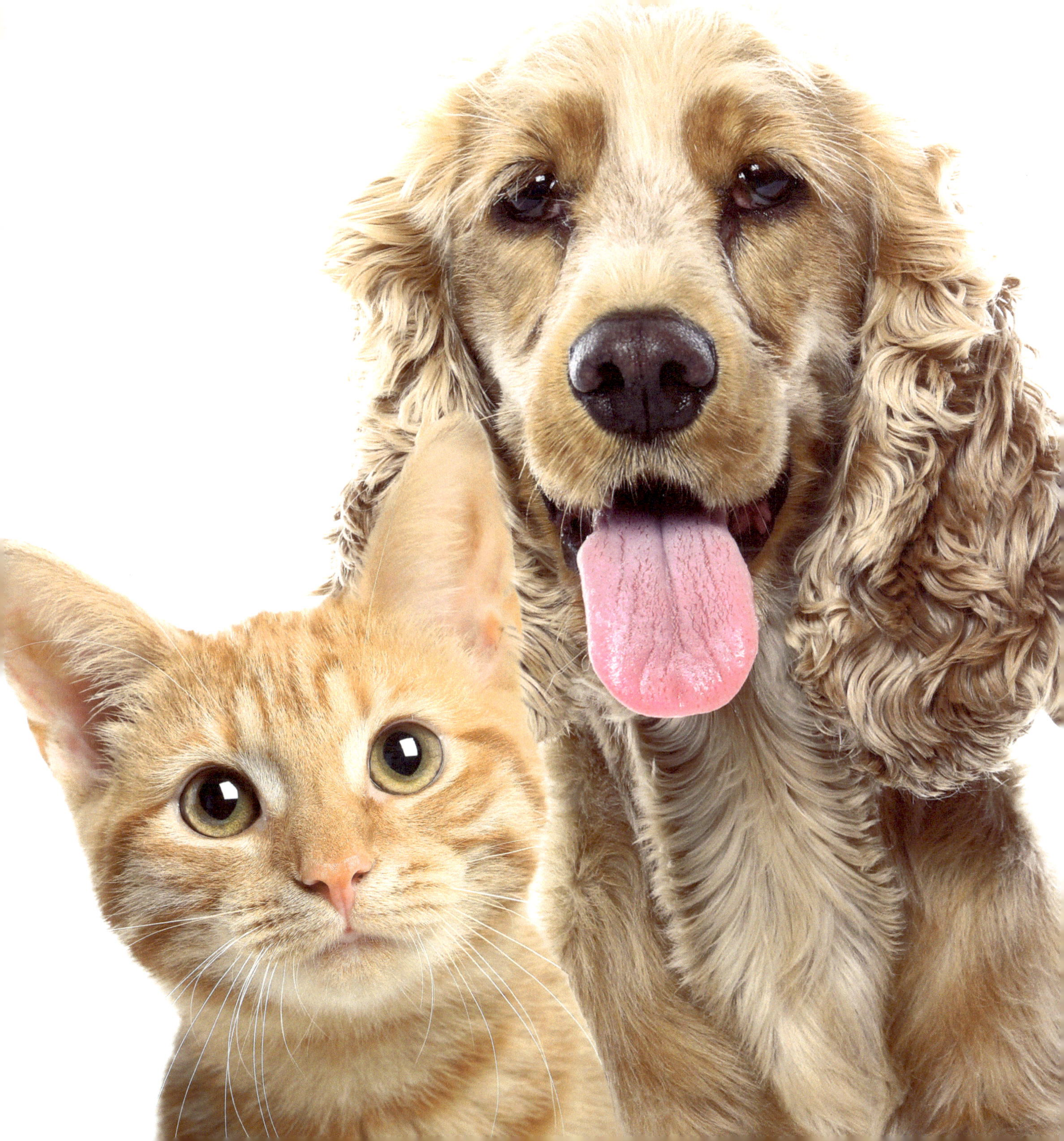

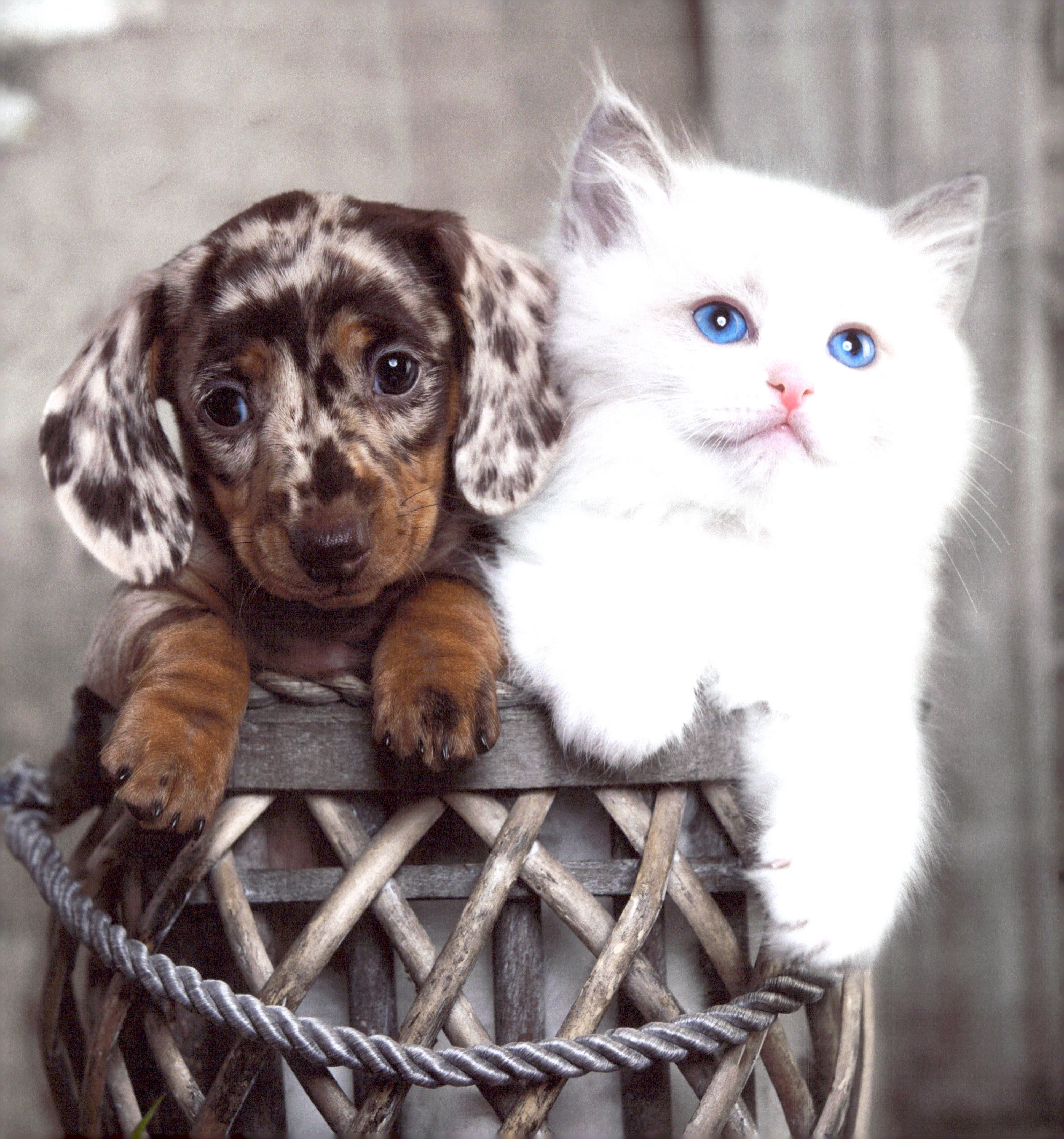

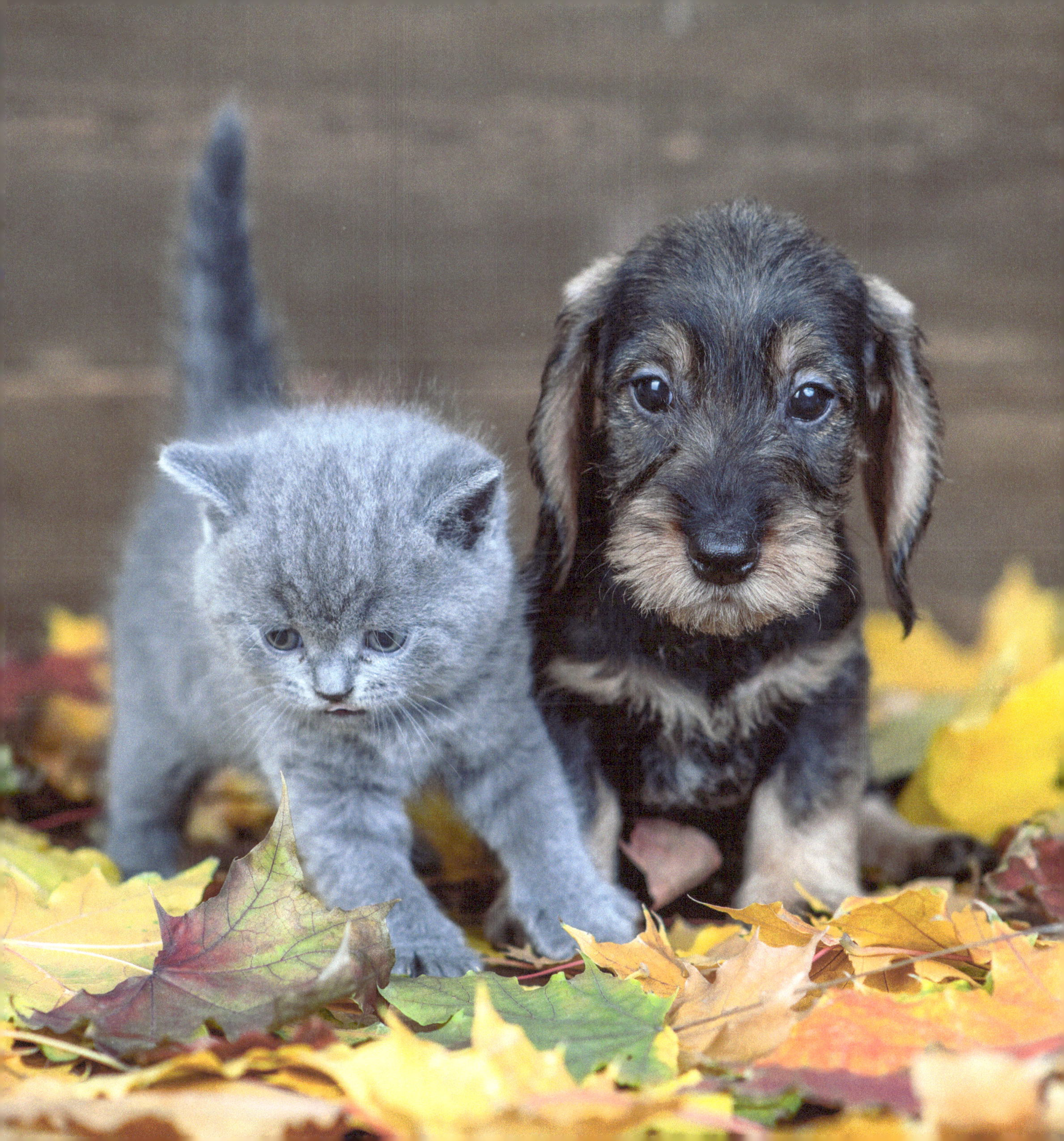

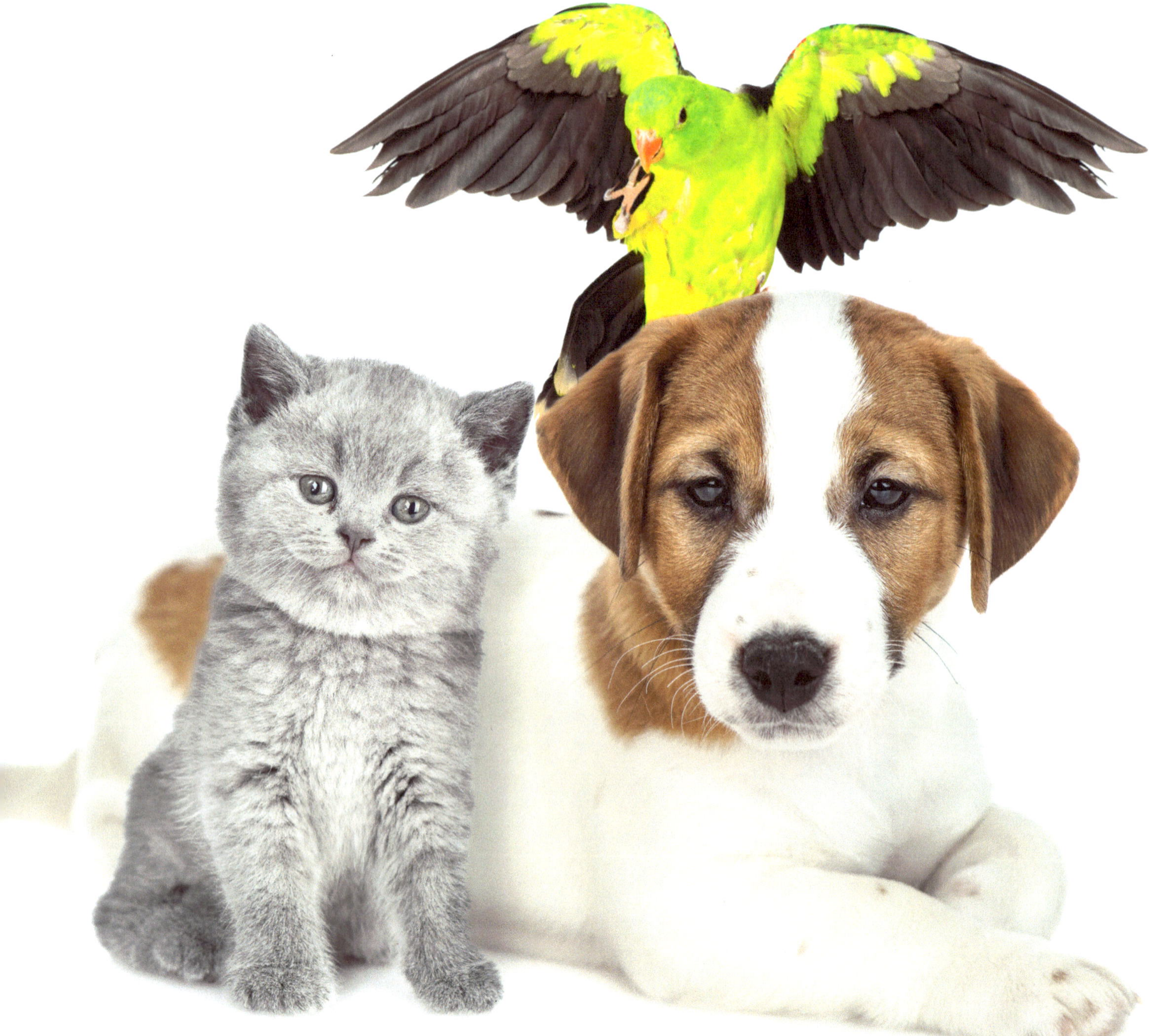

www.ingramcontent.com/pod-product-compliance
Lightning Source LLC
Chambersburg PA
CBHW041539260326
41914CB00015B/1507
* 9 7 8 1 9 9 0 1 8 1 7 0 2 *